Praise for

"Dr. Kowey has illuminated brilliantly many of the pitfalls in US healthcare today, along with their causes, using patient vignettes. Helpful guidance is offered to patients as they navigate our dysfunctional healthcare system until vast improvements in US healthcare delivery are in place."
—*Ralph Brindis, MD, MPH, MACC, former President, American College of Cardiology*

"*Failure to Treat* explains the problems with US health care and how we got here. Kowey uses stories of failure in the medical system to explain how we can advocate for our care. It will be a great addition to health humanities classes and a resource for patients who want to know more. Given the current failures of US healthcare, the book is a timely and necessary call to action."
—*Ann E. Green, Professor, Clinical Bioethics and English, Saint Joseph's University*

"This has to be required reading for EVERY medical student, physician, and patient. Kowey is a born writer and chronicler of the state of medicine. There are many practical lessons for both patients and physicians. We must take medicine back and these stories chart a beginning path."
—*Kenneth A. Ellenbogen, MD, Kimmerling Professor of Cardiology, Division of Cardiology, VCU Pauley Heart Center Medical College of Virginia/VCU School of Medicine, former President of the Heart Rhythm Society*

"*Failure to Treat* exposes the harsh reality that even the most competent and caring clinicians are often rendered ineffective by a broken healthcare system. This real-world account should shake patients, policymakers, and professionals alike out of complacency. It is a brutally honest call to fix what is failing before more lives are harmed or lost."
—*Mary Ann Peberdy, MD, FACC, FAHAC, Kenneth Wright Professor of Cardiology and Professor of Emergency Medicine, Virginia Commonwealth University*

"This inspired book is lucidly written by a distinguished physician-scientist, who is deeply committed to the health and well-being of patients. Dr. Kowey's outlook on medical care was nurtured by a giant in medicine, Dr. Bernard Lown, our shared mentor at Harvard University, who embodied his solemn commitment to treating patients with compassionate care. The critical messages are impactfully conveyed by artful storytelling drawn from real-life cases. The overall point is that medical care is a noble calling with the goal of saving lives and mitigating human suffering, and that the siren call of financial returns should not obscure the sacrosanct patient-doctor relationship."
—*Richard L. Verrier, PhD, FHRS, Harvard Medical School, Beth Israel Deaconess Medical Center*

"Provocative, thoughtful, real-life stories display the insight of Dr. Kowey's decades of experience as a preeminent cardiologist. If you care about the problems in our healthcare system and want to understand more, read this book."
—*Nancy H. Fullam, Esq., Founding Partner, Fullam and McEldrew Law Firm*

"*Failure to Treat* is not just a book, it is a wake-up call from a doctor who has spent his entire life fighting for patients, only to watch the system fail them. Dr. Kowey writes with the heart of a healer and the fury of someone who's seen too much unnecessary suffering. The stories are raw, real, and often heartbreaking. They pull back the curtain on a healthcare machine that prioritizes profits over people, leaving both patients and doctors trapped in its gears.

"I know Dr. Kowey not just as a brilliant cardiologist, but as a mentor who has guided me through my early years of attending. That is why this book cuts so deep for me. You feel his grief for a profession he loves while it is being hollowed out by greed and bureaucratic red tape. You hear the echoes of his own teacher, Dr. Bernard Lown, who warned him decades ago that medicine was losing its soul.

"This book is more than a diagnosis; it is a prescription for change. If you have interacted with the healthcare system as a nurse, provider, patient or a care giver, this book will shake you. And if you're a doctor drowning in paperwork, lawsuits, or burnout, it might just remind you why you started."
—*Ali R Keramati, MD, FACC, FHRS, Director, Cardiac Elecrtrophysiology Fellowship, Lankenau Heart Institute, Thomas Jefferson University*

"*Failure to Treat* is very well written. And Kowey's reasons for writing it, and underlying concerns, are well expressed. I am struck with the book's dedication to Dr. Lown, as well as the gist of Dr. Kowey's last conversations with him. It is further poignant that Dr. Kowey turned back to his mentor, for inspiration. I never had the privilege of meeting Dr. Lown. However, I'm sure he is proud of Dr. Kowey for his hard work on behalf of his colleagues."
—*David B. Bharucha, MD, PhD, FACC*

"The medical societies, including ours, are truly enriched by Dr. Kowey's contributions as a scientist, educator, and communicator and will have to face the dilemma of service—wherein the physician is the last advocate and protector of patients, who give their most precious possession, their health, to us."
—*Sanjeev Saksena MBBS, MD, FACC, FESC, FAHA, FHRS, FRSM, former President of the Heart Rhythm Society*

"In this outstanding treatise, Dr. Kowey, a world-recognized expert medical clinician, researcher, educator, consultant, and humanitarian, shares an insider's view with the reader that exposes the underappreciated failures within the US healthcare system that impede delivery of care to our patients at a level that they deserve and our healthcare providers desire. This book should be a must-read for all those involved not only in the delivery of medical care but also for those who control its regulations and purse strings."
—*James Reiffel, MD, Emeritus Professor of Medicine, Columbia University School of Medicine*

"As much as I've enjoyed Dr. Kowey's medical mystery novels, this book eclipses them as a must-read. I know that all healthcare providers are living this, but even they may be too close to urgent care and crowded schedules to see some of it. Certainly, lay people require insight into the bigger picture, as medicine becomes corporatized."
—*Robert Cody, MD, Former Professor of Medicine at the University of Michigan and Attending Physician, Massacheusetts General Hospital*

"*Failure to Treat* can make you a better patient. Through a series of anecdotes with explanations, commentary, and advice, it exposes the pitfalls of our health care and arms you with information to better navigate the system and advocate for what needs to be fixed.

"View this book as a Survival Guide to American Medicine."
—*Lawrence Deckelbaum, MD, Associate Head, Strategic Development, CSL Behring*

"This book effectively breaks down a complex topic. Its realistic stories not only inform, but also invite, readers to become more engaged with the subject—hopefully inspiring greater political involvement and thoughtful participation in discussions when talking to friends and family. That is the only way that things are likely to change."
—*Arnold Greenspon, former Head of Cardiac Electrophysiology at Thomas Jefferson University*

"As a primary care physician and former medical director of a national health insurance company, I can attest to the incredible dysfunction in our healthcare system described in Dr. Kowey's book. *Failure to Treat* should be required reading for anyone interested in trying to heal our diseased health delivery mess!"
—*Jay Krakovitz, MD, former Medical Director, US Healthcare*

"For centuries, the doctor-patient relationship has been a sacred ethical and moral bond between physicians and the patients who seek their advice and treatment. In *Failure to Treat*, Dr Kowey explores how multiple factors are now distorting this relationship, often to the detriment of the general public. Based on a compendium of typical patient experiences, the author explains how the complexity of healthcare in terms of evolving scientific information, technological advances and financial considerations all influence the dysfunction of our current health care delivery system.

"Each chapter concludes with advice and suggestions for measures that patients, healthcare providers and administrators, as well as government representatives can implement to restore commonsense, empathy and trust to the interactions between health care providers and their patients. As someone with 50 years of experience in clinical surgery and medical education, I plan to use the information and concepts presented in this book as I mentor the next generation of health care providers."
—*Edward Kwasnik, MD, Assistant Professor of Surgery, Harvard Medical School*

"Excellent and masterful book providing important insights into the working of our present health care system as expressed in real life stories."
—*Brian Olshansky, MD, Professor Emeritus and Electrophysiologist, University of Iowa*

"This book is a wake-up call to the lay public regarding the deterioration of our healthcare system despite the incredible scientific medical advancements that have occurred over the last 4 decades."
—*Irving M. Herling, MD, Emeritus Professor of Medicine, Thomas Jefferson University and the University of Pennsylvania*

"In *Failure to Treat*, Dr. Kowey lays bare the myriad issues that plague, and may ultimately bring down, the US healthcare system. It is eye-opening, not only for the lay public who will inevitably need to seek healthcare, but also for physicians and others who work within the system."
—*Ronald Haberman, MD, Electrophysiologist and Pharmaceutical Industry Consultant*

"I just read the introductory chapter, and you have literally taken the words out of my mouth."
—*Stephen C. Vlay, MD, FHRS, Professor of Medicine, Stony Brook University*

"Dr. Peter Kowey has had a long career advancing the state of medicine to enable us to live longer and be healthier. With a messianic voice, he writes about the impediments preventing modern medicine from doing better in his new book, *Failure to Treat*. With a frustrated pen, he writes about onerous paperwork that often hides diagnostic reality; the grinding industry of malpractice lawyers that can take an inordinate amount of cash from medicine, drive doctors into early retirement, and cause doctors to burden the system with procedures based on fear of getting sued; the explosive growth of medical bureaucrats making medical decisions to the detriment of patients; the deadly game between insurance companies trying to limit excessive procedures and those demanding procedures that can result in denial of common sense prescriptions; the games of the pharmaceutical industry, and much more.

"The reader is taken through a maze of patients who did not receive the benefits of modern medicine because of a myriad of transgressions. A series of actual health incidents is presented, followed by an explanation, a

commentary, a conclusion, and advice for patients. Dr. Kowey has seen it all, and from all sides of the medical equation."
—*Stephen Lee Crane, Former President and CEO, Pavilion Press*

"This excellent book is a must-read for patients as well as those who have not yet experienced the health care system. It should also be required reading for federal and state legislators to fully understand the current state of the health care industry—and an industry it has become. I have seen the evolution of the advances in clinical health care, as well as the devolution of the business aspects of the medical profession, which has led to the health care crisis that Dr. Kowey so clearly describes."
—*Judith Mackarey, healthcare attorney*

"In *Failure to Treat*, Dr. Kowey details the shortcomings of the American healthcare in a series of compelling patient stories. Practicing physicians and patients alike will recognize the situations. Kowey, an accomplished cardiologist and writer, makes a passionate, convincing case for urgent reform of the business of medicine."
—*Roger M. Mills, MD, FACC, former Professor of Medicine University of Florida; former Vice President of Medical Affairs, Scios Inc.*

"Through real-life vignettes, Dr. Kowey carefully and thoughtfully describes issues facing patients and medical providers today, highlighting why it is imperative that each of us has an advocate when navigating our healthcare system. A must-read for medical professionals and patients alike."
—*Cynthia H. Richards, MD, MBA, former Medical Director, Pharmaceutical Research and Development*

"With these heartbreaking stories of medicine gone wrong, coupled with a clear-eyed analysis of the often non-medical reasons why, Dr. Kowey brilliantly shows the perils of modern healthcare. *Failure to Treat* lays bare systemic failings while affirming medicine's timeless values: listening, caring, and never losing sight of the patient. The book provides an unflinching portrait of systemic failure that every healthcare provider will recognize. In capturing both the daily frustrations and the enduring ideals of good medicine, Kowey makes plain that the situation is desperate—and demands urgent attention."
—*Kristen Patton, MD, FACC, FAHA, FHRS, Professor of Medicine, Division of Cardiology, University of Washington*

"The stories in *Failure to Treat* deliver frightening and essential insights for us all. The cases presented reveal the troubling evolution of our health care system—from one centered on patient welfare and protection to one increasingly driven by the financial interests of insurance companies and for-profit health care entities.

"What makes this book especially valuable, though, is that in addition to exposing the systemic failures that undermine both access and quality of care, Dr. Kowey offers clear, practical recommendations—from how patients can better navigate the system to how we might improve medical education, reform physician compensation models, and restore integrity to clinical care. *Failure to Treat* is both an exposé and a roadmap—a book that empowers patients, challenges policymakers, and speaks directly to health care professionals who still believe in medicine's moral core. It's a vital read for anyone who cares about the future of American health care."
—*Liza Seltzer, former Execute Vice President and Chief Operating Officer, ACI Research*

"Peter Kowey, MD is the Sherlock Holmes of modern medicine. *Failure to Treat* is written for patients and families, and describes how medicine and health care impacts everyone's wellbeing."
—*David E. Behrend, financial consultant*

"The twenty case stories are real-life examples that bring to the forefront the wrong direction that healthcare has taken in this country today. These stories pertain to me both professionally and personally. Over thirty years in the pharmaceutical and medical device industry, I've worked hand-in-hand with physicians, nursing staff, office personnel, and administrators. I have seen and felt the decline in the relationship between physicians and their staff with industry representatives like me. Physicians have little time, and administrators guard against industry influence. Under these circumstances, this book brings value and perspective to patients who are making crucial healthcare decisions."
—*Gerald Mayza, pharmaceutical representative*

FAILURE TO TREAT

How a Broken Healthcare System Puts Patients and Practitioners at Risk

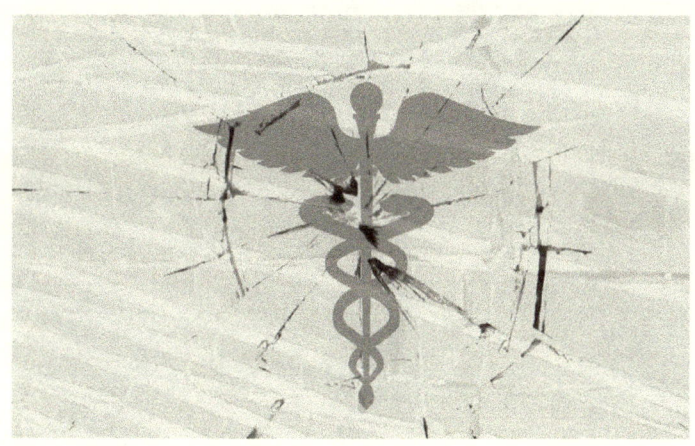

PETER KOWEY, MD

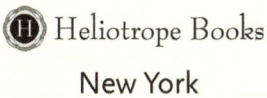

Heliotrope Books
New York

Copyright © 2025 Peter Kowey, MD

All rights reserved. No part of this book may be reproduced or transmitted in any form or by any means, electronic or mechanical, including photocopying, recording or by an information storage or retrieval system now known or hereafter invented—except by a reviewer who may quote brief passages in a review to be printed in a magazine or newspaper—without permission in writing from the publisher.

Heliotrope Books LLC
heliotropebooks@gmail.com

ISBN 978-1-956474-69-5
ISBN 978-1-956474-70-1 eBook

Designed and typeset by Naomi Rosenblatt with AJ&J Design

DEDICATION

This book is dedicated to my mentor, Dr. Bernard Lown. A Nobel Peace Prize Laureate and internationally renowned scientist, Dr. Lown's greatest achievements were at his patient's bedside, where he made it his habit to heal hearts and to mend souls.

Much of this book emanates from conversations I had with Dr. Lown in his final months. By exposing every part of the scandal that medicine has become, I hope that healthcare providers can begin the process of resuscitating our beloved profession, and our patients can more successfully navigate their way to better health.

Disclaimer: The twenty vignettes in this book represent a fusion of several real cases, but all people and place names are entirely fictional. To enhance the reading experience, details such as conversations and memories have been added but are not meant to be an actual account. Any resemblance that the characters in this book may have to real people is unintentional.

All of the opinions stated in this book are mine alone, and do not reflect the views of the institutions where I have trained or worked, my employers, colleagues, or patients.

CONTENTS

Prologue   15

Story 1: Medical Insurance Companies Do Not Care About You
    • Ms. Ping and Dr. Xavier   21

Story 2: Healthcare Screening for Fun and Profit • Mr. Jay   34

Story 3: The Medical Malpractice Disaster • Mrs. Apple   43

Story 4: The Rise of the Administrators • Mrs. Lopez   51

Story 5: The Electronic Medical Record: Boon or Bane?
    • Mrs. Francis   62

Story 6: Precertification Doesn't "Certify" Anything
    • Mrs. Dowd and Dr. Thom   73

Story 7: Direct-to-Consumer Advertising and Other Drug Company
    Nonsense • Mrs. West and Dr. Shah   85

Story 8: Technology for its Own Sake • Mr. Lee and Dr. Gold   98

Story 9: Regulatory Failings and the Billion-Dollar Alternative
    Medicine Mess • Mr. McCabe and Dr. Nuff   111

Story 10: Physician Burnout is Real and Really Bad for Everyone
    • Mr. Han and Dr. Robb   122

Story 11: It's All About the Money: For-Profit Outpatient Procedural
    Centers • Ms. Nell and Dr. Bank   135

Story 12: Physician Reimbursement and Perverse Incentives
 • Mr. East and Drs. Silver and Wynn   146

Story 13: The Medical Education Fiasco • Mrs. Uler and Dr. Yeats   157

Story 14: Acquisition Mania and the Private Equity Mess
 • Mr. and Mrs. Epps and Dr. Herr   169

Story 15: Affiliated Healthcare Professionals Are as Good as Doctors. Really? • Mrs. Hernandez and Nurse Practitioner Antman   181

Story 16: Research Data and How to Manipulate Them
 • Mr. Quinn and Dr. Vijay   190

Story 17: Diversity and Inclusion: Do We Need a VP or a Dean for That?
 • Mrs. Engle and Dr. Isaac   204

Story 18: Those Big Centers Love to Tell You Just How Great They Are
 • Mrs. Lynch and Drs. Keats and Wolf   213

Story 19: Medical Clearance or How to Blame Somebody Else
 • Mr. Coyle and Drs. Wynn and Singh   227

Story 20: Fragmentation of Care: Doctor, Who Are You Again?
 • Mrs. Anders and Dr. Orly   237

My Overall Conclusion   249

Acknowledgments   257

Glossary   259

Author Bio   262

PROLOGUE

"We have to ask ourselves whether medicine is to remain a humanitarian and respected profession or a new but depersonalized science in the service of prolonging life rather than diminishing human suffering."
—Elisabeth Kubler-Ross

I have been a physician for five decades. I came to medicine as a complete innocent. No one in my extended family had made it to college, let alone professional school. I was inspired by the family doctor we visited when I was in grade school. An elegant and caring man who wore a nice suit and a bow tie every day, he had a beautiful office with gentle dogs to pet in the waiting room. Without a single office helper, he dispensed care in a way that made my family feel comforted and healed at the same time. So, when my relatives would ask me what I wanted to be when I grew up, I answered "a doctor," completely unaware of what that meant or what it would take to get there, including the financial resources that my hard-working blue-collar parents simply didn't have.

I graduated from high school as an immature and naïve boy. After a difficult journey through college and medical school, during which I nearly gave in and quit, I chose to pursue a career in cardiology, inspired during my internship by two young physicians who were technically gifted and fiercely dedicated to dispensing superb medical care to all their patients. I remember calling them in the middle of the night to come to the hospital to help the house staff care for sick patients with life-threatening cardiac problems. They brought not only breathtaking expertise, but also patience and a calm demeanor that immediately put all of us, nurses, young doctors, and patients, at ease.

One of those mentors and now a fellow author, Dr. Barbara Roberts, convinced me that pursuing fellowship training at her alma mater would be to my great benefit. How right Barbara was, for not only did I find a discipline that I loved intensely, but also several teachers who spent time helping to steer me to my final professional destination, cardiac electrophysiology. Principal among my superiors at Harvard was Dr. Bernard Lown. Trained by the master clinician, Dr. Samuel Levine, Dr. Lown was the consummate physician, spending hours at the bedside, using his skills in physical examination as well as history taking, extracting critical information from the patient, including the psychological triggers that so many times were the cause of manifest cardiac disease. His patient rounds and clinical conferences were a revelation to me, and his example instilled in me an ability to relate to my patients, to care for the person and not the disease, and to measure success not by cure, rarely attained in medicine, but by return to a high level of function and an improved sense of wellbeing. He taught us how to preserve patient hope and to avoid words, phrases, even gestures or voice inflections that might rip asunder the therapeutic bond. Maintaining hope and cautious optimism were paramount. I remember how Dr. Lown lashed out at a house officer who told a patient's wife that the blockage in her husband's coronary artery was a "widow-maker," a term that frightened her terribly. He was also the first person to point out to me that sitting down to talk to a patient was a poignant sign that the doctor was not in a hurry, and that whatever the patient had to say had great importance. He emphasized the importance of addressing patients by their surnames, never using first names without the patient's insistence, as a sign of respect. There was no such thing as diversity training; all patients were to be treated with the same level of caring and concern without question or exception. Violation of that principle was simply not tolerated and a reason for summary dismissal from the training program.

Ironically, it was Dr. Lown's own terrible experience as a patient at the end of his life that started me on the path to writing this book. He complained bitterly about fragmentation of care, the slavish dependence on technology, the shoddy nursing care, and the cavalier attitude of his physicians and surgeons that made each of his hospitalizations torture. All of this was particularly galling to Dr. Lown who had dedicated his entire life to compassionate care. Dr. Lown chided me for not being enough of a public advocate for our profession and our patients as he was. After he died, I vowed to accept his challenge and tell the story of how medicine as a profession is in jeopardy of falling from its lofty place in our society to a job on the assembly line, widgets replaced by patients.

I have spent my medical career caring for patients with cardiac rhythm abnormalities, and, as an academic, carrying out research, teaching and writing. I have appreciated my profession for what it has afforded me: an opportunity to lift the burden of disease from another human being's shoulders and allow that person to live a life unencumbered by the worries and doubts that disease engenders. There is no greater privilege than to be admitted into the lives of other people, not only to learn about their disease, but, more importantly, to become privy to personal and cherished aspects of their existence. I will be forever grateful to all the people who inspired me, trained me, and worked with me to make sure that the patients I touched would have nothing but the best care.

Paying it forward, I have spent a significant part of my career in medicine as a teacher. I have instructed medical students, residents, fellows and physicians in practice for many years and have taken great pleasure from that experience. Teaching has allowed me to extend my reach, and to positively influence the care of patients by the example I have set for my students, and through the lessons I have tried to impart. I have also been a researcher for many years, having conducted and supervised clinical trials. As with teaching, I believe that my work in clinical research has had a ripple effect by improving the care of patients with cardiac rhythm problems.

I have told you, the readers, about myself so you can understand that writing a book which takes the medical field to task has been the most difficult undertaking of my professional life. Herein, I lay bare several problems that interfere with a physician's ability to deliver the highest standard of care to his or her patients. The motivation to do so has been my frustration as I have watched my beautiful profession assaulted, torn down and thoroughly disrespected by people who have no idea what being a doctor really means. I believe I owe it to my colleagues to write a book that strikes back at the ignorant, the vile, and the manipulative people who have ruined a tradition of healing to which we have literally dedicated our lives. I also want to address the anger so many of my patients have voiced after being mistreated by insurance companies that deny tests and procedures or being overcharged for therapies that they desperately need to feel better and live longer.

This book is not intended to be a medical text. I have used language that should be interpretable by lay people and professionals alike, avoiding jargon and medspeak that patients find obtuse and sometimes desultory. I deliberately did not list literature references to support my opinions. None of the facts in this book are controversial. They have been stated many times in various publications by erudite people, and we all know them to be true. In addition, I didn't want to burden the reader with a myriad of references they would never use and that would only divert attention from the fundamental principles that I am anxious to convey. I have sought to emulate physicians like Sam Levine and Bernard Lown, who made the case of what our profession is supposed to be, and where it has failed, using allegory and commentary in their own manner. Finally, I have made light use of statistics for similar reasons and because, as Dr. Lown was fond of saying, if you need statistical treatment of data to make them persuasive, perhaps they are not important enough.

The other significant part of my career has been creative writing, an interest I cultivated in college and returned to years ago. Storytelling is an ancient art that has enormous educational value. Dr. Lown himself was a master storyteller and frequently used vignettes to drive home critically important clinical lessons. The enthusiastic reception my novels have received from medical professionals provided me with the idea of using storytelling to deal with the many issues that have plagued medicine.

What follows is a series of short stories, which were synthesized from hundreds of patient cases in which I participated during my many years of clinical, research, regulatory and consulting activities. Every story reveals a part of what is wrong with our healthcare system, and how patients and healthcare providers are being harmed by obstacles to good care that are frequently generated by greed. As noted in the book's disclaimer, none of these stories come from a particular institution or from any one patient or patient family. In addition, fictional details have been added to preserve anonymity, to make the stories readable, and to illustrate important patient care issues.

I did not write this book with a hostile or destructive intention. Neither doctors nor patients have anything to gain from turning medicine into a mushroom cloud. Furthermore, I will emphasize that most healthcare providers are highly principled, well-intentioned people who truly have patients' best interests at heart. My own experiences as a patient have reinforced my high opinion of providers at all levels, and of the ancillary staff who work hard for relatively meager wages to make our offices, clinics and hospitals run as well as they do. Those kind people treat their patients as they would their family because, in doing so, they believe they are making this world a better place for all of us. It is a minority of practitioners who have chosen greed over principle and have besmirched the reputation of our professions. But it is their egregious actions that capture the attention of the media, especially when cases come to light in high-profile litigation. Instead of banishing these villains from our profession, we, their colleagues, compound the scandal by turning a blind eye.

I would also emphasize that there is no place for politics in this discussion. Although I criticize many of the policies put into place by our federal government, neither party has done much of anything to remedy the current situation. The last several administrations have made small improvements, but we are left with a gaping wound for which a band-aid simply will not suffice. In addition, most of the needed changes will not be enacted at the federal level but rather by the states, which means that pressure on local legislators will be our most productive strategy.

I have yet another important goal for this book. Despite all its problems, I continue to advise young people to consider healthcare professions as a career choice. How succeeding generations will practice will be different, and that is to be expected. However, I want future doctors and nurses and other healthcare providers to make their career decisions with their eyes wide open. There can be nothing as discouraging as investing money and years into education and training only to find that the goal so ardently pursued is corrupt and no longer worthy of the struggle to achieve it.

I truly hope this book helps all of us to refocus on what makes medicine so wonderful and diminishes the distractions of profit and power that have led to the sad stories told herein. I welcome dialogue with healthcare professionals, patients, payers, administrators, and lay readers because only through the process of self-examination and external critique will we improve a broken healthcare system to which people needing care entrust their very lives. To that end, I invite interested people to access my website: **peterkoweyauthor.com.** There you can share your views and stay current as I regularly update and create video and print material to address new developments in the struggle for better medical care for all.

Story 1: Medical Insurance Companies Do Not Care About You

"When it is about your health, the decision maker should always be a doctor, not an accountant." —Chuck Schumer

NARRATIVE

Ms. Ping was a 33-year-old Asian woman who played first violin for a major metropolitan orchestra. She was a child prodigy who ascended from a prominent music academy to the junior orchestra and then to the full ensemble in record time. She was married to another musician, and they lived in a city condominium close to the music center where they both performed regularly. Because of their heavy travel schedules, the couple decided to hold off on having children for a few years.

Ms. Ping was in good health and kept herself in excellent physical condition with regular exercise at her condo's workout facility. She had no family history of cardiovascular disease and, though she occasionally had a marijuana cigarette with friends or a couple of martinis on weekends, she did not abuse drugs or alcohol and took no prescription medications.

Then, one morning, while running on the treadmill, the machine alarmed, informing her that her heart rate was very high, more than 180 beats per minute. She quickly stopped the machine and stepped off, but it took several minutes for her heart rate to return to normal. Although she had ignored heart skipping in the past, over the following weeks she had more frequent episodes of severe palpitations, feeling the gradual onset of a regular and rapid heartbeat along with mild shortness of breath and dizziness. The symptoms occurred at rest or with exertion, but if she stopped and took several deep breaths, the palpitations would ease a bit faster.

Through her care portal, Ms. Ping messaged her primary care doctor, who advised a visit and an examination, the findings of which were negative except for a resting heart rate of 100 beats per minute. The electrocardiogram confirmed sinus tachycardia (a fast but normal heart rhythm). Otherwise, that test was normal as were the results of a full battery of blood tests. Most importantly, Ms. Ping had normal thyroid function, was not anemic, and had no electrolyte abnormalities to explain her elevated heart rate. Given no evidence of heart or other disease, her doctor advised a period of watchful waiting to see if her symptoms improved on their own before ordering more cardiac tests.

Ms. Ping's symptoms didn't improve but worsened over the next month to the point that she stopped exercising and had to miss several orchestra practices and a few performances. Her primary care doctor finally referred her to a cardiologist, and he was savvy enough to choose a cardiac rhythm specialist, Dr. Xavier. On her initial visit with Dr. Xavier, Ms. Ping carefully explained her symptoms, highlighting their gradual onset and long duration with slow and partial resolution. Once again, the physical examination and electrocardiogram showed an inappropriately elevated heart rate and nothing more. An electrocardiogram and echocardiogram were likewise normal, showing no evidence of heart disease of any kind.

Dr. Xavier recommended further testing to look for more unusual diseases of the endocrine system, like an overactive adrenal gland, which could cause a fast heart rate, but those test results were negative, too. At that point, Dr. Xavier recommended a 14-day continuous, outpatient cardiac monitor to determine exactly what Ms. Ping's heart rhythm was when she had her most intense symptoms.

Ms. Ping had several rather severe episodes of palpitations over those two weeks, some when exerting but many others at rest, and some even awakening her from sleep. She wore her monitor compulsively, removing it only when she showered, so she hoped to finally get a diagnosis and treatment plan when she returned for her follow-up appointment with the cardiologist.

Ms. Ping was not disappointed. Dr. Xavier was able to tell her that her symptoms correlated with sinus tachycardia. In essence, for unclear reasons, periodically Ms. Ping's normal electrical system would simply speed up, causing her heart to race. The diagnostic term was "inappropriate sinus tachycardia," because the increase in heart rate had no apparent cause. Although not common, it is a well-described entity that mainly affects women between 20 and 40-years-old. The condition causes palpitations and dizziness, but usually is not associated with severe heart disease and does not damage the heart. The primary reason to treat it is to get rid of symptoms that interfere with normal function.

The news was reassuring to Ms. Ping, who was anxious to begin treatment. The cardiologist told her that the process would be one of trial and error. She would prescribe a drug known to reduce heart rate and ramp up the dose to tolerance. If that drug didn't work, she would try another or even a combination of agents that lowered the heart rate by different mechanisms. She would continue to monitor Ms. Ping's heart rate carefully so as not to slow it too much, or to drop the blood pressure, as many of the drugs that slowed heart rate were wont to do.

Dr. Xavier began with a beta-blocker from a class of drugs designed to lessen the effects of adrenalin on the heart, thus reducing the normal heart rate and blood pressure. Unfortunately, the process of discovering the right drug for Ms. Ping did not go quickly. Despite trying three different preparations of beta-blocker at an optimized dose, Ms. Ping's heart rate remained elevated, even though her blood pressure was abnormally low, and she felt lethargic.

Dr. Xavier then tried two different calcium channel blockers at high doses without much improvement. Like beta-blockers, these drugs also have a direct effect on the sinus node, the pacemaker of the heart, but they too lowered Ms. Ping's blood pressure to the point that she now could no longer play the violin—let alone participate in orchestral performances. She became agitated and depressed, desperate to find a solution after so many weeks of uninterrupted symptoms and failed treatments.

Dr. Xavier told Ms. Ping that there was one more drug they could try, called ivabradine. It was a relatively new drug that had a selective effect on the sinus node, and thus the heart rate, and had been shown in several studies to be effective for patients with inappropriate sinus tachycardia. Ivabradine was approved in several European and Asian countries and was marketed in the United States, but not for arrhythmia. It had been approved by the United States Food and Drug Administration to treat patients with refractory heart failure, in whom a reduction in heart rate was beneficial for optimizing cardiac performance. It was not widely used because it was expensive, and there were several other drugs for heart failure that were generic and thus cheaper.

Knowing that ivabradine was available, and after establishing that Ms. Ping had a prescription plan through the company that provided health insurance for the orchestra, Dr. Xavier ordered the medication for Ms. Ping at a low starting dose. But when she went to the pharmacy to pick-up the drug, she was told that the insurance company would not approve payment, so she would have to pay out-of-pocket. Desperate, Ms. Ping agreed, but was shocked when she was presented with a bill for $800 for a one-month supply.

Ms. Ping called Dr. Xavier to find out what she could do to obtain ivabradine at a more reasonable price. Dr. Xavier gave Ms. Ping samples to use for a few weeks while her office sorted through the payment issue with the insurance company. Ms. Ping had a marvelous therapeutic effect from ivabradine, with an almost complete resolution of her symptoms. She was overjoyed and grateful.

While this treatment trial with free samples was under way, Dr. Xavier asked her nurse practitioner to call the insurance company to determine what paperwork was needed to get the drug for Ms. Ping for chronic use. This phone call was the start of a three-month saga, during which the nurse practitioner and the cardiologist spoke with or emailed several individuals at the company to convince them to approve payment for what the company considered an "off-label" use. That is, the company paid for the drug for patients with heart failure, but since Ms. Ping did not have heart failure and ivabradine was not approved in the US for inappropriate sinus tachycardia, payment was denied.

There was one more chance. Dr. Xavier was finally granted permission to have what is called a "peer-to-peer" conversation with an insurance company physician. When they finally connected, the company doctor began by admitting she had been trained as a psychiatrist and didn't have expertise in cardiology. However, she told Dr. Xavier that she had researched the ivabradine issue and convinced herself that the evidence to support its efficacy for inappropriate sinus tachycardia was limited and inconclusive. The company had no intention of paying for "experimental therapies."

Dr. Xavier was prepared. She started out by telling her "peer" that Ms. Ping had had a very good response to the drug samples. She was then chastised by the company doctor, who reminded Dr. Xavier that dispensing samples for off-label indications was unethical and illegal. Dr. Xavier ignored the barb, knowing full well that using samples in such a way was common practice and sensical. She pointed out that several other countries had granted approval for this indication and that her interpretation of the literature was much different. Dr. Xavier offered to send the company doctor copies of some relevant articles, including one that Dr. Xavier herself had co-authored. Furthermore, Dr. Xavier argued that Ms. Ping was desperate. She had tried and failed every other known medical treatment and was disabled by severe symptoms.

Dr. Xavier did not win the day. Two weeks after the call, the insurer issued a final judgment of no payment. Dr. Xavier told Ms. Ping that she would continue to appeal the decision, but she was not optimistic. Ms. Ping would have to pay for the drug, find a new insurance company, or consider an ablation procedure.

Ms. Ping was not poor by any means, but she knew that she couldn't afford to pay for ivabradine indefinitely. Her health insurance was through her employer, the orchestra, and so finding and paying for another insurance plan was not an option. Before deciding what to do next, she wanted to know about ablation.

Dr. Xavier explained the procedure to Ms. Ping, including the need to insert catheters into vessels in her groin to be threaded into her heart. The ablation catheter would be placed in the region of the sinus node and hooked up to a radiofrequency generator with the intention of cauterizing the tissue responsible for the fast heart rhythm. Dr. Xavier told Ms. Ping that ablating the sinus node to cause it to fire at a reduced rate was tricky business. First, no one in the world had extensive experience with sinus node ablation, given the rarity of Ms. Ping's disorder. Also, there was no consensus as to how many radiofrequency lesions or burns should be administered via a catheter placed in the sinus node region to diminish its function, and how best to assess whether the procedure was successful. There was also a significant chance of damaging the node so much that it no longer functioned at all, in which case a pacemaker would be required to support her heart rhythm for the rest of her life.

Ms. Ping was in a quandary. She and her husband decided to seek a second opinion with a rhythm specialist at another university hospital. This cardiologist was not nearly as pessimistic about the ablation procedure as Dr. Xavier had been. He said he had performed dozens of the procedures with remarkably good success. The better news was that he would be able to use "creative coding" for the ablation, so her insurance company would pay for the procedure if she decided to go in that direction. "One and done," he said, "and no more expensive drugs with side-effects."

It shouldn't be difficult for the reader to figure out what happened next. Ms. Ping had the ablation procedure with the second specialist, and the insurance company paid for it, as he predicted. The insurance company also went on to pay for the permanent pacemaker that Ms. Ping needed after the ablation because her sinus node had been fried into oblivion. The damage quickly became clear in the recovery area where her heart rate dripped into the 20s, and she nearly lost consciousness. She was rushed back into the electrophysiology lab where she had a temporary pacemaker inserted into her heart. When her own heart rate didn't come up to normal, a permanent dual-chamber pacemaker was placed a few days later.

In exchange for palpitations and dizziness, Ms. Ping was faced with a lifetime of pacemaker management, including frequent visits, generator changes and the inevitable deterioration of the pacemaker leads that would require reoperations for repair. The insurance company that refused to approve treatment with ivabradine paid not only for the ablation and the pacemaker implantation but also for years of pacemaker management, the cost of which would easily top seven figures.

CASE EXPLANATION

Appropriate sinus tachycardia is a reactive increase in heart rate usually caused by an increase in metabolic demand, such as exercise or fever. Inappropriate sinus tachycardia is a very uncommon condition, but, as with Ms. Ping, it can cause disabling symptoms. It is highly disconcerting to feel your heart begin to race without any provocation. The reason is not known but one theory is that it is caused by up-regulation of an ion current that is unique to the sinus node, called If or the "funny current." Ivabradine is the only drug that selectively blocks the funny current and thus slows the sinus node without affecting other parts of the electrical system and not depressing cardiac function or lowering blood pressure, as beta-blockers and calcium channel blockers do. Ms. Ping's rhythm disorder did not respond to approved medications but ivabradine worked for the few weeks she used samples. So why wasn't the drug made available for her?

Drug development is a complex business. Bringing a new chemical entity to market is enormously expensive, usually costing billions of dollars. Because patents have a limited life, pharmaceutical companies have a finite amount of time to recover their development costs and then to make a profit.

If a newly approved drug is used in many patients, the price may be high but somewhat affordable for most patients. But for those drugs approved for an "orphan indication," that is, for a very small target population, the price is usually much higher. Though heart failure is a common disease, when ivabradine was approved for heart failure, it was with the expectation that it would be used in a small subset of patients, those in whom a high heart rate was thought to be particularly detrimental to cardiac function. Inappropriate sinus tachycardia, the other indication for ivabradine, is so rare that the sponsoring company didn't waste time and energy trying to obtain a secondary approval for it in the US. Thus, ivabradine was left with a high price tag and no FDA approval for its off-label use in desperate patients, and thus little or no motivation or imperative for the insurer to pay for it in Ms. Ping's case.

Without a drug treatment option, Ms. Ping's only realistic alternative was ablation. Here again, she did not have good fortune. Sinus node ablation, despite the second opinion physician's enthusiasm, is a poorly conceived procedure with an inadequate knowledge of nodal anatomy and physiology to instruct the operator about how and precisely where to place radiofrequency lesions. Many electrophysiology laboratories have abandoned the procedure altogether, especially those outside of the US because there, patients have access to and are well served with ivabradine treatment. Ms. Ping stumbled onto one of the last few zealots clinging to the idea that sinus node ablation could be carried out safely and successfully. Unfortunately, in Ms. Ping's case, he was wrong.

As a result, Ms. Ping would be faced with life-long pacemaker maintenance. Pacemakers, like all machines, are not fully reliable. A particular issue is lead durability. Pacemaker leads, the wires that connect the device to the heart muscle, are engineered to work for months to years, not decades. They are used, in almost all cases, in elderly patients with a limited life expectancy. Lead failure is a potentially catastrophic event. Not only is the patient left without an adequate heart rate to sustain blood pressure, but procedures to extract and re-insert leads are not inconsequential. These problems, together with generator depletion and replacement, are a heavy burden for a relatively young and previously healthy person.

COMMENTARY

Have you watched television commercials for medical insurance companies? They all contend that they care about your health. To some extent, they do because having a large stable of healthy subscribers for whom healthcare costs are low is essential for their financial success. It is the population of old and sick people on whom they must spend the most money. For those high-end users, the gambit is to pay as little as possible. One way of doing that is by denying medical insurance for people with "pre-existing conditions," which, in effect, kept sick patients out of the risk pool. That strategy was rendered illegal in the Affordable Care Act, thankfully, although experts warn that it may be resurrected by the current administration as a favor to the insurance industry that donated heavily to the winner's campaign.

If government regulators are going to allow "non-profit" insurance companies to routinely operate with a large revenue margin, we must expect that they will be motivated to pursue another money-saving tactic, denying payment for drugs and procedures as they now do in upwards of a quarter of claims. Non-payment is justifiable under some circumstances, such as when there are no data to support off-label usage. But this begs the question as to who, exactly, makes these determinations? Insurance companies may depend on advice from clinical guideline committees to establish appropriateness of treatment, but they are not bound to do so. State insurance commissions supposedly provide oversight of payment issues, but rarely deal with individual case decisions, and almost never scrutinize payment for drugs for rare diseases. Frustration with dealing with a deaf and poorly regulated medical insurance industry led to the highly publicized and brutal murder of a company executive in December 2024, which was unabashedly applauded by millions of angry insurees.

As in Ms. Ping's case, appealing insurance company decisions is torture for patients as well as healthcare providers. The process begins with a phone call or email to a clerk, usually yielding nothing since that person will recite policy from the company manual. Several more calls are needed to get to a nurse or nurse practitioner who may have more knowledge but is not empowered to make a payment decision. Hours of staff and provider time are spent on these preliminary calls. They are never answered promptly, usually require several minutes to hours on hold, and rarely provide a definitive answer.

Ultimately, a "peer-to-peer" conversation is required. When finally connected, the insurance company physician at the other end of the line may be from a different specialty but profess to be willing to listen to the patient's advocate doctor before deciding how to proceed. Whether that conversation is fruitful and succeeds in getting the medication for the patient is unpredictable. Quoted success rates for peer-to-peer appeals are in the range of 50 percent.

To make matters even more complicated, Medicare has become entangled in insurance company decisions because of a relatively new business model called Medicare Advantage. When the Medicare law was passed, to assuage private insurers, it was determined that Medicare would pay 80 percent of the costs of medical services such as office visits and hospitalizations. The other 20 percent would need to be covered by some form of private insurance, sometimes referred to as Medicare Supplemental Insurance. Dealing with multiple insurers placed a heavy burden on elderly Medicare patients, so insurance companies were allowed to offer plans by which they would pay a patient's total healthcare costs while collecting the Medicare portion. The patient needed to sign up with one of the Medicare Advantage plans but would only pay one monthly premium. The problem has been that despite playing with Medicare money, Medicare Advantage insurers pursue the same ruthless tactics of requiring pre-certification for many procedures and then denying care, again about 20 to 25 percent of the time. The current administration has proposed forcing all Medicare patients into Advantage plans, in essence privatizing medical care for all seniors.

Medicare has also refused to negotiate drug prices for the elderly to keep them in a reasonable range. Medicare patients are responsible for a significant percentage of the cost of their medications depending on how much they have spent on co-pays in any 12-month period. This has led to the dreaded "donut hole" period when patients must absorb all or nearly all the cost of their drugs. The Biden administration began a process by which costs of common but expensive drugs might be capped for Medicare recipients. It took only a half century to move that idea forward and the program is now in jeopardy with the arrival of a new, industry-friendly healthcare administration. Though Donald Trump has paid lip service to reducing drug prices and issued executive orders, no meaningful policies to control costs have been put into place.

Perhaps the root of the drug pricing and accessibility problem is the lack of synchronization between drug approval and drug pricing. The Food and Drug Administration (FDA) is charged with reviewing new drug applications and expanded labelling of existing drugs based strictly on evidence of effectiveness and safety in comparison to a placebo. The FDA does not require a positive comparator study in which the new entity is compared to an existing product that is considered the standard of care. Furthermore, neither the FDA nor its many expert advisory committees are permitted to consider cost or pricing in their deliberations about approvability and labeling of new drugs and devices. Thus, cost-effectiveness is not part of the drug approval process.

By comparison, in Europe, the cost of medication is regulated. In those countries, the decisions to approve and to price are carried out concurrently. Only drugs that produce a significant advantage in safety or efficacy compared to conventional treatment can command a premium price. In the US, the same free market principles that govern common commodities pertain. There are no limits on what pharma companies, buttressed by their powerful lobbies, can charge for their products. Free-market pricing necessarily works to the detriment of patients in desperate need of effective and frequently live-saving treatment.

Recently, attention has been focused on yet another reason for high drug prices: the exorbitant fees charged by Pharmacy Benefit Managers, unregulated agents who bring drugs from the drug manufacturers to retail pharmacies and hospitals. Their huge profits have come as a direct consequence of overcharging drug manufacturers and pharmacies, which in turn raise their prices to maintain a profit margin. Guess who loses in that scenario.

Refusal to pay for important drugs and procedures pales in comparison to huge coverage gaps in preventative treatments. The most glaring is underpayment for dental and eye care. Despite compelling evidence that poor dental hygiene is directly responsible for cardiovascular events, and that poor vision causes depression and loss of autonomy in seniors, most of the cost of preventing and treating common maladies like gum disease and glaucoma are borne by patients. Medical insurance typically covers a small percentage of the real cost of care, forcing providers to charge less and patients to pay more than the insurance companies. Many if not most employers no longer offer vision or dental care as an employment benefit and, if they do, a significant contribution by the employee is required. Once again, our legislators have failed to enact legislation to provide fundamental health services for the old and poor, the result being that only the wealthy can afford to take good care of themselves. If you want to talk about health equity, this would be a very good place to start the conversation.

CONCLUSION

Two separate problems led to Ms. Ping's conundrum. First, her health insurance company denied payment for a drug that was, for her, clearly safe and effective. As we will see in the next vignette, health insurance companies are powerful and have been able to stay in business despite all the harm they cause. Consider that thousands of patients lose access to their practitioners any time a health insurance company refuses to negotiate their rates with a healthcare system, and that there is little anyone can do to prevent this catastrophe.

The United States Congress has been stubbornly resistant to the idea of a single healthcare payer. "Medicare For All" has not had enough support for passage, in large part because the private health insurance lobby is incredibly strong and active. Thus, we still have a patchwork of payers, and, though many call themselves "non-profit," they are very much in the business of accumulating capital.

As in several areas of medicine, the opportunity to profit from disease management necessarily produces inequities. Many people are simply unable to afford health insurance and require public assistance available through Medicaid, which has traditionally restricted access to expensive drugs. The passage of the Affordable Care Act (Obamacare) provided some relief, but many exchanges struggle to stay afloat in the currently adverse political environment and simply don't have the capital to pay for costly drugs and procedures. The chances of a Medicaid patient gaining approval for a colonoscopy are virtually nil. And if it is bad now, wait until deep cuts in Medicaid come into play.

Recent events have focused public attention on the nefarious practices of medical insurance companies. Unfortunately, it took a deadly attack on a healthcare insurance executive. Around the same time, idiotic reimbursement policies came to light such as not paying for anesthesia care if an operation takes longer than expected to complete. We can only hope that the media that has covered these events so extensively continue to keep us informed of obvious injustices unless and until real changes are enacted.

The second problem leading to Ms. Ping's predicament was the ridiculous prices that are charged for medications in the US. Big Pharma's powerful lobbies have prevented reform. If anything, drug prices have risen, especially when those products are developed for rare or very serious diseases. There seems to be no lack of funds to pay for absurd television ads. How much less could drugs cost if hundreds of millions of dollars weren't wasted on advertising to a naïve public?

Insurers have pushed back hard against negotiating prices with Medicare on the premise that they need a large profit to fund research for new therapies, dodging the question of why US patients pay orders of magnitude more money for common medications than any other citizens of first world countries.

This story has dealt with a patient who had reasonable insurance and yet couldn't break through to obtain a costly medication that likely would have made her feel better and obviate the need for a costly and risky procedure. How ironic that the insurance company, which denied the drug, would be saddled with the costs of an ablation procedure, a long and complicated hospitalization, temporary and permanent pacemaker implantation, and a lifetime of device maintenance after the procedure they did approve went sideways.

There are no easy solutions. Importing drugs from Canada and other foreign countries could be a good idea, but free of regulation, many of those drugs are counterfeit, often worthless placebos packaged as real drugs, and newly imposed tariffs will make drug importation even more problematic. Enforcing price control and demanding evidence of cost-effectiveness would work, but that would require new laws. A Congress that can't stop mass murders of children by passing an automatic weapon ban is unlikely to take on Big Pharma lobbies. And so, once again, the American public suffers because of the greed of businesspeople who pay tens of millions of dollars to tell you in TV commercials that they really do care about you.

PATIENT ADVICE

It is incumbent on patients to be highly engaged and informed as they make decisions about their healthcare coverage. This is no easy task. It is difficult to understand how much medical procedures cost, and how much patients will be responsible for paying out of pocket. Exactly why an insurance company only has to pay a small portion of some astronomical sum that a hospital charges for a common operation is difficult to discern. Nonetheless, insurees cannot become so angry that they purchase a weapon and gun down the head of a healthcare insurance company on the street. Instead, they need to channel their frustration and elect and pressure legislators to protect their right to good and affordable healthcare with a wholly transparent price. They need to vigorously oppose cuts in funding for Medicare and Medicaid services, and pressure lawmakers to eliminate our patchwork and hopelessly complicated payment system. The holy grail is a universal healthcare plan that grants access to good doctors and hospitals for everyone at a reasonable price.

In the meantime, choosing an appropriate and affordable health insurance plan, especially for seniors, is a daunting task. It needs to be approached carefully and after consultation with an expert who can explain the advantages and drawbacks of the several available options. Issues to consider are freedom of choice of physician, participation by local healthcare facilities, deductible amounts and co-pays, and payment for drugs, vision, and dental care.

We can only hope that our leaders will eventually awaken to the crisis and the need for wholesale reform of our broken medical insurance system, and the need for greater regulation of the pharmaceutical industry. But as my mother used to say, "Don't hold your breath."

Story 2: Healthcare Screening for Fun and Profit

"A vigorous five-mile walk will do more good…than all of the medicine… in the world." —Dr. Paul Dudley White

NARRATIVE

Mr. Jay was a 50-year-old Caucasian man who kept himself in generally good health. He exercised regularly and limited his diet to what he considered healthy foods. He worked long hours at his garage as a mechanic to support his wife and two teenage children. Risk factor management was particularly important in Mr. Jay's case because his father died of a heart attack at 60-years-old and his older brother was diagnosed with coronary artery disease at a similar age. His primary care doctor was satisfied with his overall health, including his blood pressure and weight, his cholesterol and blood sugar levels. He took vitamins and fish oil and didn't smoke or use drugs. He liked to have a few beers with friends on the weekend but was careful to moderate his alcohol intake.

One day, while scrolling through the local news on his phone, Mr. Jay saw that a company was conducting a weekend cardiovascular screening at a nearby high school gym under the auspices of his local community hospital. Mr. Jay clicked on the link and made an appointment, figuring that it couldn't hurt to get tested to make sure his heart and blood vessels were as healthy as they could be. He was informed that the cost for the tests was $400, which included a detailed explanation of the tests and a report reviewing in detail any observed abnormality. Mr. Jay was told he would need to pay for the tests on arrival with a credit card and could submit the receipt to his insurance company for reimbursement. The testing company stipulated that it couldn't guarantee payment by a third-party insurer because the tests were not being carried out for a specific diagnosis.

Mr. Jay arrived on time and was excited to see how many of his neighbors and friends joined him, and how well organized the event was. He was escorted to a separate tent for each of his five tests: an electrocardiogram and 10-minute heart rhythm recording, an echocardiogram to look at his heart chambers and valves, a carotid ultrasound to determine if there were any blockages in the vessels that supply blood to his brain, an abdominal ultrasound to look at his aorta, and an arterial Doppler study to make sure he had adequate blood flow to his lower extremities.

The testing went quickly, and Mr. Jay was on his way home within an hour, pleased with the experience and looking forward to getting the results of his tests, due in a few days by email. As promised, a message arrived with a 10-page PDF attachment that began with a disclaimer that the test results should be considered preliminary and should not be acted upon until consultation with his private physician.

Mr. Jay began to review the results and was excited to see that almost everything came out fine. He was pleased that his electrocardiogram, blood pressure, echocardiogram and peripheral artery tests were unremarkable. The only abnormal finding was disease in his left carotid artery, with an obstruction estimated at about 60 to 70 percent. The report explained that this degree of blockage may be associated with a high risk of stroke and that he should consider further testing and consultation with a specialist. The company gave him the name of one such specialist, who happened to be a surgeon employed by the sponsoring hospital.

Mr. Jay called his family doctor. The call back took a couple of days during which Mr. Jay became more and more stressed and agitated. When he returned the call, the family doctor agreed that a consultation with a vascular specialist would be a good idea and gave Mr. Jay the name of an experienced vascular doctor at the university hospital whom he knew and trusted. When an appointment with that person couldn't be arranged for four months, Mr. Jay decided to see the hospital-based surgeon whom the testing company had suggested.

Mr. Jay was able to make an appointment for the following week and went to the office with his wife. He brought along his test results. The specialist was a nice and relatively young man who took a brief history and listened to Mr. Jay's carotid arteries. Though he didn't hear any turbulence with his stethoscope, he told Mr. Jay that the test interpretation was probably correct. He explained that this degree of carotid disease put him at a substantial risk of a stroke. He told Mr. Jay to add 81 mg a day of aspirin to the statin he already took, and advised Mr. Jay to strongly consider having a procedure to relieve the blockage. The choices would be an operation known as an endarterectomy or a catheter procedure to essentially ream out the atherosclerosis and place a stent. Mr. Jay was told that the operation might be his better choice. The specialist was a surgeon who happened to do endarterectomies.

After discussion with his wife and family doctor, Mr. Jay decided to have the surgery. The procedure was scheduled for two weeks later at his local hospital. He had the usual pre-operative testing that once again confirmed his overall good health. He arrived at the hospital, was prepared by a nurse and an anesthesiologist, and brought into the operating room where he was put under. When he awakened, he had mild discomfort over the left side of his neck and was relieved to see his wife standing on the right side of his bed, smiling down at him. He tried to tell her how happy he was to see her but couldn't form the words, nor could he use his right hand or arm to reach out to her.

CASE EXPLANATION

Mr. Jay suffered an intra-operative stroke, a known and feared complication of carotid surgery. The left side of Mr. Jay's brain had been deprived of adequate blood flow for at least several minutes during the procedure. Since he was under anesthesia, his loss of function was only detected when he woke up in the recovery room. A neurological consultation was called. Physical findings suggested that a large part of Mr. Jay's brain was affected, a finding confirmed by a CAT scan and an MRI of the brain.

Why did the stroke happen? There are several possible reasons. It could have occurred because debris from the lipid buildup in his carotid artery showered into his brain. During manipulation of the carotid artery, the vessel might have spasmed, causing the brain to be deprived of blood for a long time. The stroke also could have been the result of the surgeon damaging the vessel and causing it to shut down. How much the stroke could be attributed to bad luck versus lack of surgical skill would never be known, although Mr. Jay later learned that the nice young surgeon who operated on him had performed only a handful of endarterectomies since he finished his training.

I am frequently told by patients that they would rather die than suffer a large stroke and I understand that feeling completely. Mr. Jay was an active, vibrant and productive individual whose life would never be the same after his stroke. After aggressive rehabilitation and good care he was able to recover some of his strength and speech, but he couldn't return to his employment and would be permanently disabled, reliant on his wife for many of his activities of daily living.

COMMENTARY

There is little information to support mass screening for almost any disease. Testing for conditions such as breast, prostate, or colon cancer may have merit but only when those tests are selected, ordered, and supervised by a personal physician who is fully acquainted with the patient and his or her medical history. The doctor and the patient must be convinced that the information to be gleaned is essential for the patient's wellbeing, and that the testing will be carried out by competent individuals at certified, experienced facilities. Most importantly, there needs to be a high "pre-test probability" so that an abnormal finding is more likely to be a true positive rather than a false positive result.

None of that was true in Mr. Jay's case. He had no idea who performed his trailer tests, who interpreted them, or how to properly place the results in perspective. Consequently, he agreed to have carotid surgery without precisely understanding its benefits and risks. He didn't know that operating on asymptomatic patients with non-critical carotid artery disease is, at best, controversial. Depending on the surgeon's skill and experience and the nature of the lesion in the artery, the incidence of stroke with the procedure may be higher than the risk of leaving the vessel alone and taking medications. Instead, Mr. Jay was referred to an inexperienced surgeon and to a hospital that were incentivized to recommend and perform surgery that in the end proved catastrophic.

Incidental health screenings are ubiquitous, and cardiovascular testing is the most notable and popular. The purveyors of mass screening appeal to the "worried well," who are usually affluent, white-collar, upper-class, and upper-middle-class people who may have some vague reason for concern but who are not having a problem. In Mr. Jay's case, his principal concern was his family history. Granted, his family history made him more aware of the need to exercise, control his weight and do all the things to preserve his cardiovascular health. The mistake he made was believing that a potentially risky procedure would increase his chances of remaining alive and event-free.

Mr. Jay was surprised by the results of his tests and appropriately so. No one suspects or wants to learn that the vessels that supply blood to the brain are diseased. However, what Mr. Jay didn't have was an informed and sympathetic doctor who could explain to him that arterial disease is ubiquitous, and that 60 to 70 percent lesions are common and not life-threatening. Millions of people in the United States have some degree of atherosclerosis and never have a clinical event. When blockages are discovered incidentally, medical treatment is intensified with drugs to inhibit platelet activity and lower cholesterol to very low levels. That is the most important treatment to prevent the plaque in the artery from rupturing and causing a large stroke, or a transient ischemic attack (TIA) or mini stroke.

Perhaps even worse than a result that is difficult to interpret is the abnormal finding that no one was looking for. Medical people call them "incidentalomas," abnormalities on an imaging test that might be benign but could also be cancer. The good news about such a finding is that an unsuspected cancer may be caught while still in a curable phase. The bad news is that, much more frequently, the exact nature of the finding cannot be determined by imaging alone, which mandates an invasive procedure to find out the patient has a malignancy. While very few such lesions are cancerous, the upheaval visited on the patient and family is monumental. Not only does the patient have to wait for a biopsy procedure, but it is then days and sometimes weeks until the pathology report is available. Exactly why it takes so long to examine a surgical specimen has never been adequately explained to me or my colleagues by the administrators responsible for that process. They appear to be as deaf to patient suffering in this scenario as they are in other clinical situations. In any case, patients who go through this agonizing experience learn the hard way not to have testing done unless it is absolutely necessary.

By going to an unknown testing center, Mr. Jay violated one of the most important rules in medicine: do not fragment care. When patients consult with multiple doctors or visit unfamiliar facilities, they invite disaster from lack of effective communication. Hospitals advertise to entice patients to move their care to a new facility for their own financial interests, unconcerned about the importance of continuity. Patients need to know that leaving one's usual health orbit should be undertaken only when the added expertise of a specialist is necessary and not to be found anywhere else.

Most egregious in Mr. Jay's case was that a local hospital sponsored the mass screening for its own selfish reasons. The hospital put its reputation on the line for an unregulated testing company because, whether by agreement or by a tacit understanding, the health screening company was expected to refer patients with positive findings to specialists employed by the hospital. This ensured that office consultations and procedures would fall to them. The more positive test results, the better for the hospital—never mind the agony patients experienced waiting for the results of further imaging or biopsy. This arrangement should give the reader a good understanding of how competitive healthcare institutions are for patient revenue, and the extent to which they will go to keep their volumes up and the revenue flowing.

As you will see in subsequent stories, medical insurance companies can be quite difficult to deal with, for both physicians and patients. However, for all their faults, these organizations spend a good deal of time, energy, and money trying to determine which medications, tests, and procedures are the most likely to keep their beneficiaries out of the hospital and event free. When they believe that there is no benefit to a test or operation, they refuse to pay for the service. Such is the case for mass cardiovascular screenings. First, there is little or no assurance of reliability. The results generated by trailer testing of the kind Mr. Jay had are almost never subjected to any kind of quality control, which is a requirement at hospital laboratories and facilities.

Most importantly, there are no data that patients can derive benefit from random screening. Even worse are the downstream consequences of positive or overly interpreted tests. Ironically, though the insurance company denied payment for the screening, Mr. Jay's insurance company did pay for the carotid surgery because the consulting surgeon certified in the medical record that Mr. Jay was at a high risk of stroke, even though the data to support that conclusion were weak at best.

A prime example of mass testing driven by inappropriate concern is athlete screening. It is true that young people can die suddenly while engaged in sporting activities, but the incidence is low, lower than the risk of being struck by lightning. However, when these tragic events occur, they attract media attention and prompt outcries for more cardiac testing for young athletes. While there is value to a thorough history and physical examination for all children, there is little evidence that applying a battery of expensive tests is worthwhile.

Not all children and adolescents who die suddenly are athletes or participating in athletic events at the time of their death. The rationale for screening athletes only is therefore difficult to understand. Most importantly, the probability of heart disease in a group of active young people who have no symptoms is extraordinarily low. Therefore, for every true positive test in this population, there may be tens or hundreds of false positives. These misleading results cause havoc emotionally for the athlete and his or her family. At best, a false positive result leads to a battery of costly follow-up studies; at worst, it may lead to an inappropriate decision to bar the child from participating in a sport they love or for which they may have particular talent.

Finally, this case raises several questions about the adequacy of informed consent. Though the consultant surgeon certainly was not negligent in his recommendations, was Mr. Jay fully aware of the possible consequences of the procedure before consenting to it? Was he advised of what the medical literature had to say about the relative benefit of medical treatment versus the risks of an invasive procedure for the treatment of patients like him with asymptomatic carotid artery disease? Did he understand the relative benefit of medical treatment versus an invasive procedure and the risks of each? If he were asked in retrospect, and if he could answer, Mr. Jay likely would probably say that he was not fully aware of the inadequacy of the data that led the surgeon to recommend a procedure that ruined his life.

CONCLUSION

There are several valuable lessons to be learned from Mr. Jay's case. I counsel young physicians to have a firm idea about what they will do with the results before they order any test. This principle is certainly applicable in Mr. Jay's case. Finding out that he had carotid disease was valuable in that it should have helped him be more careful about controlling factors that would impact his cardiovascular risk. Though he couldn't change his genetics, he could take measures to improve his health and his chances of maintaining good health.

However, using the results of that random screening to justify a potentially risky operation was unwise. Careful consideration of the consequences of any intervention is so important that, depending on the circumstances, gathering a second opinion before any major surgery is a good idea, especially when recommended by a physician who is not known to you.

"If it ain't broke, don't fix it," is an adage that applies in Mr. Jay's case. Our quick-fix culture frequently compels us to look for easy solutions to complex problems, of which atherosclerosis is certainly an example. Consider that even with our current state of knowledge, we simply don't understand when or why a plaque in a coronary or carotid artery will rupture and hemorrhage, occluding the vessel and causing a heart attack or stroke. Given our limited knowledge of the biology of the most common arterial disease in creation, categorical recommendations about interventions to improve prognosis are presumptuous and as likely to result in dire outcomes as to help.

In short, the lesson to be learned is that excellent patient care requires a thoughtful and individualized approach by a learned and compassionate healthcare provider, relying on hard scientific data whenever possible. Knowledge of the probability of disease before ordering tests is paramount. Only by strict adherence to this rule can we avoid calamities like Mr. Jay's.

PATIENT ADVICE

Doctors are highly educated people who generally have the patient's best interests at heart, but sometimes struggle to communicate just how beneficial a treatment may be, and how best to balance that benefit against the risks of a drug or procedure. One useful way of interpreting the relative value of a medical procedure is to ask about a measurement called *number needed to treat*. By measuring the absolute difference in efficacy between two therapies in a clinical trial, it is possible to describe how many patients will need to be subjected to a treatment for one patient to be benefited. For carotid operations in patients who have never had a stroke or TIA (mini stroke), at least a hundred surgeries would have to be carried out to prevent one death or major stroke. Given the hazards associated with the surgery, a truly informed patient, hearing that, might opt for medical treatment alone, especially if the risk of the operation was greater than one percent.

The best way to access good and reliable healthcare is through an excellent primary care physician. Specialist-hopping, independent of your doctor's recommendations, fragments care and will place you in peril. Even worse, participating in mass screenings, or responding directly to media advertisements will inevitably lead to frustration and worry, if not a calamity. In the best of circumstances, real medical problems will not be solved. Worse, you might be exposed to a substantial risk of unnecessary and, in some cases, downright dangerous procedures or medications with a negligible chance of prolonging your life or improving its quality.

Story 3: The Medical Malpractice Disaster

"Never go to a doctor whose office plants have died." —Erma Bombeck

NARRATIVE

Mrs. Apple, a 55-year-old African American widow, lives by herself on a pleasant city street. Today, we find her lying on a stretcher in the middle of the hallway of her local emergency room. Her 30-year-old daughter, Maisha, who brought her to the ER eight hours ago is seated in a folding chair next to the head of the stretcher, exhausted from waiting around all day for any kind of guidance or diagnosis. Mrs. Apple's splitting headache, for which she came to the hospital, is finally beginning to ease, but not because of any treatment she has received from the ER staff. In fact, the only thing that may have helped a little was the ice pack she had brought from home, now still in place, but long gone warm.

Mrs. Apple is a headache veteran, having experienced typical migraines for years. She has learned that if she can respond quickly, severe headaches gradually abate with rest and a couple of ibuprofen capsules. This headache had come on strong and ibuprofen didn't work. Mrs. Apple's primary care doctor, who no longer takes emergency calls, had prescribed a variety of medications over the years that were too expensive for her to purchase and use regularly. She had let the latest sample of a "miracle remedy" expire in her medicine cabinet when it didn't work any better than ibuprofen.

Emergency room visits were only occasional and fortunately, as she got older, the spells were not as long or as severe. Until today, that is. This headache had persisted for three hours, prompting her to call her only daughter for assistance and a ride to the local emergency room for relief.

As usual, the ER was crazy busy. Mrs. Apple had to sit for three hours in the waiting room until Maisha was able to convince the triage nurse that her mother's condition was serious and worsening. Since all examination rooms were occupied, Mrs. Apple was placed on a stretcher that was then parked in a hallway with a flimsy curtain drawn around it, preserving little privacy. After a nurse recorded her vital signs, a nurse practitioner came by to talk to Mrs. Apple and her daughter, and to do a perfunctory physical examination, the results of which she declared to be "normal," without any neurological deficits. She left to confer with the doctor in charge of the shift. About an hour later, the nurse practitioner returned to collect blood samples, and to tell Mrs. Apple that she would be transported to radiology soon for some tests. When Maisha asked what tests had been ordered, the nurse practitioner replied, "brain imaging."

Another hour went by before a nice elderly man in a blue jacket came to transport Mrs. Apple to the X-ray department. He told Mrs. Apple that he was a hospital volunteer, a retired lawyer in fact, and that part of his service was to move patients around the hospital for testing and so on. Mrs. Apple asked the man several questions about the tests she was going to have performed, and he provided more detail than the nurse practitioner who had ordered them. Mrs. Apple was going to have a CAT scan and an MRI of her brain to find out what was causing her continuing and excruciating and not yet treated headache.

Despite her claustrophobia, Mrs. Apple persevered through the imaging tests and was returned to the ER hallway where she and her daughter waited for the results. What they didn't know is that the tests were going to be read by a radiologist who was off-site, and in fact not even in the western hemisphere. They also did not know that Mrs. Apple was being evaluated by a nurse practitioner and a supervising physician who had only recently been named in a malpractice case that was eerily like her own.

Two more hours elapsed, during which no one came to her bedside. Maisha finally corralled a harried nurse and asked when her mother might receive medication for her lingering headache. She was told that it would be dangerous to prescribe anything until the doctors "ruled out an intra-cranial catastrophe," a term unfamiliar to them but to Mrs. Apple sounded ominous and frightening.

The ER adventure finally came to a denouement when a neurology resident came to see Mrs. Apple a few hours later. After repeating her neurological examination, he was able to tell her that all her tests had been negative for a stroke or a hemorrhage, and that Mrs. Apple's headache was most likely a migraine. When Mrs. Apple pointed out that she had told the nurse practitioner that she had a history of migraine and that this ache in her head, though prolonged, was totally typical, the resident could only shrug and reassure her that the testing had been necessary to determine the most appropriate treatment. Maisha asked him, "What would you recommend?"

"Since your headache has let up, I think a couple 200 mg tablets of ibuprofen should do the trick," the resident replied. The resident would have the nurse bring the medication to Mrs. Apple straight away.

That translated into another 30-minute wait, after which Mrs. Apple was told to get dressed. Remaining behind the screen while trying to put on her bra and blouse wasn't easy, but, when finished, she headed to the front desk where she was given twenty pages of information and instructions, the most ridiculous of which was a reminder to return to the ER immediately if her symptoms recurred.

CASE EXPLANATION

Unfortunately, Mrs. Apple's ER adventure was not unusual. Patients who visit emergency facilities in the United States routinely wait for hours before they are seen and evaluated. They frequently have a variety of unnecessary tests before being treated, in many cases, inadequately. The problem is a consequence of incidental and fragmented care caused by the inaccessibility or unavailability of physicians who know the patient and can initiate care confidently. That issue, as well as overly zealous testing, is addressed in later stories in this book. But Mrs. Apple's tale is important because it exposes one of the most insidious and vicious problems that plague medical care in America: the doctor's fear of being sued.

Why did Mrs. Apple have such a costly and failed ER visit? She had no way of knowing that her nurse practitioner and supervising physician had been sued for malpractice. In that case, a middle-aged man with a recurrent headache had been evaluated and discharged from the very same ER a few months before, only to be found dead at home hours later. Autopsy showed an intracranial hemorrhage—that is, bleeding into his brain. Because his symptoms had been so typical of his usual stress-related headaches and eventually relieved with Tylenol, and because his neurological examination had been negative, he didn't receive brain imaging.

The ER staff was faulted and deemed negligent by an aggressive medical malpractice attorney. An emergency room physician from a small community hospital affiliated with an Ivy League university was hired as an "expert consultant" for the plaintiff. The shill was a gifted actor who played well in front of a lay jury. He painted the defendant doctor as either a numbskull or a villain for not having ordered a CAT scan and for sending the patient home without a "proper evaluation for a brain hemorrhage." The case was still in litigation and would be for years. The plaintiff's family had rejected a $4-million-dollar settlement offer and intended to request punitive damages against the doctor and the nurse practitioner.

Mrs. Apple's ER physician was not going to let something like that happen to him again. And neither was his co-defendant nurse practitioner. If a patient came to their ER with a headache, they were going to be imaged no matter how typical the presentation or how normal their physical examination. End of story. Mrs. Apple just happened to be in the wrong ER at the wrong time, seen by profoundly psychologically wounded, defensive professionals.

This circumstance resulted in the very long and frustrating ER visit for Mrs. Apple and an $11,000 bill for lab tests and imaging as well as a $2500 consultation fee for the neurologist who had sent his resident to evaluate and dispose of the patient. All of this when all Mrs. Apple really wanted and needed was a medication, other than what she had at home, to make her migraine headache go away.

COMMENTARY

I wrote my first novel, *Lethal Rhythm*, to call the public's attention to the plight of sued healthcare providers. The book may have increased awareness of the issue, but there has been no substantive malpractice reform. Caps on awards for pain and suffering that had been enacted in several states to limit enormous non-economic awards did not gather enough momentum to prompt federal legislation, and many of those state laws have since been repealed. The malpractice bar has brought enormous pressure to bear on state legislators not only to remove those caps, but to reinstate the ability to sue doctors in any venue that is plaintiff-friendly, rather than in the locality where the alleged malpractice occurred. In Pennsylvania, that plaintiff-friendly venue is Philadelphia where juries are notorious for astronomical verdicts, far more than reasonable economic recovery. The plaintiff bar has also effectively blocked establishment of arbitration panels, which would obviate the need for courtroom drama, and thus significantly reduce the trauma that doctors suffer when accused of being negligent.

The US malpractice system has fostered the emergence of attorneys who are eager to prosecute cases that have the potential to win large awards, of which their share is exorbitant by any standard. Think about the fact that plaintiff malpractice attorneys are some of the wealthiest people in our communities, having extracted hundreds of millions of dollars from the healthcare system by collecting nearly half of the awards made to patients and families who have been harmed. Those billboards and television advertisements you see for personal injury attorneys are expensive ,as is their lifestyle. The money to pay for all of that comes directly from the healthcare system with absolutely nothing to show for it.

The escalating cost of malpractice insurance is the direct consequence of an overactive plaintiff's bar as well as the exorbitant fees charged by defense firms who stubbornly continue to argue cases that have no merit. In addition, our system does not provide a solution to remove repeat offenders. Clearly incompetent doctors who have had multiple judgments against them continue to practice and harm unwitting patients.

The malpractice system harms many people, including patients like Ms. Apple. But does it have to be this way? Is there another way to provide compensation to the innocent victims of real malpractice? The answer is a resounding yes. Other developed countries have put into place arbitration panels, consisting of knowledgeable doctors, lawyers, judges, and advocates, who rapidly and without bias assign monetary awards based on economic loss. Physicians who repeatedly come to judgment are appropriately censured but healthcare providers who have simply made a mistake are not whipsawed in a way that persuades them to leave the profession, to kill themselves, or, at best, to forever order unnecessary expensive tests in their own defense.

Patients have asked me why doctors react so strongly to being sued. After all, isn't that what malpractice insurance is for? First, malpractice insurance may, under some circumstances, not fully cover the defendant's liability. Punitive damages, as threatened against the ER doctor in our vignette, are usually exorbitant and if awarded by the court, are not covered at all by malpractice insurance.

Furthermore, it is difficult to convey to a non-physician what being sued in a malpractice case feels like. These are people who have entered medicine to help patients and to make their lives better. During their medical training, they were not schooled in any way regarding medical malpractice and what it means, let alone how to navigate through a case. Now, despite what might have been their best efforts, a patient has died or been harmed in an unintended and possibly unforeseen way. There might have been a mistake or an error in judgment for which the physician is intensely sorry. Doctors, like everyone else, make mistakes. We have learned that errors in medical care are far too common, and the consequences can be dire. But to meet the legal standard of malpractice, the physician needs to be declared reckless and intentionally negligent in an open court of law, judged by a jury that has little or no medical expertise. Information about the public trial frequently makes its way to the lay media to the physician's intense embarrassment.

The psychological harm this public accusation causes cannot be discounted. And the fact that litigation may go on for years, with endless interrogatories and depositions as a prelude to an excruciating court experience, makes the entire experience painful beyond description. And even more maddening is the potential for a physician to be dragged into a case in which he or she had little participation, in the lawyer's efforts to ensnare as many insurance policies as possible to bolster the size of the verdict or settlement.

I have had the opportunity to defend physicians in malpractice cases in which I have been convinced that they were neither careless nor negligent, but rather the unfortunate participant in an inevitably bad outcome. I have watched these caring people harden before my eyes, transformed into bitter, defensive cynics, no longer capable of giving compassionate care to anyone. They come to believe that every patient they see, no matter how young or old or friendly or hostile, might become an adversary, intent on taking them to court and wreaking havoc on their lives. Many contemplate and some attempt suicide.

Not only have I defended physicians, but I have been sued myself on three occasions. This is not surprising in itself, since nearly all doctors in high-profile specialties get sued during their career. In each of my instances, after several months or years of agony, I was dismissed from the case, which is also not an atypical outcome in the American malpractice gambit. I can say, without exaggeration, that since those lawsuits, I no longer have any encounters with patients during which the thought of a potential malpractice action doesn't enter my decision making. I fear that it has become part of the fabric of my practice, a subliminal response that prompts me to order tests that I know are unnecessary but will serve to buttress my defense should the patient come to some kind of adverse outcome, and I am sued. How many times has a fellow or resident asked me why I ordered a test in a clinical situation in which it was clearly unnecessary, only for me to have to answer embarrassingly that they were right, and I was intentionally "covering my ass."

There is also the jeopardy of "curbside consultation." Woven into the fabric of medical practice is the ability to "pick the brain" of a senior associate or an established expert about a particularly thorny clinical problem over the phone or in a hospital corridor. Patient identity is not disclosed, and there is no assumption of responsibility for proffered advice. Sadly, despite providing sage advice with no compensation, physicians have been enjoined in litigation regarding the care of a complex patient they never saw or evaluated and who ultimately fared poorly.

And then there is the guideline conundrum. Professional organizations publish hundreds of these documents, which are meant to help doctors manage common diseases. Guidelines can be based on solid clinical data, but studies have demonstrated that at least 75% of what guideline committees instruct doctors to do is not predicated on data from randomized clinical trials, but rather on weak evidence or even just expert "opinion." Nevertheless, despite the fact that guidelines are not the same as a standard of care, plaintiff attorneys use guidelines like clubs, bludgeoning defendant doctors who may not have walked the straightest of paths, ignoring the fact that each patient's case is different and may require a unique approach. Trial lawyer associations are currently lobbying to make guidelines the only metric by which malpractice is measured, intentionally excluding expert testimony that is critically important to place those guidelines in proper context.

CONCLUSION

The need for substantive malpractice reform is real and urgent. Worthless malpractice litigation harms every individual associated with the healthcare system except for the unprincipled attorneys who reap lavish and undeserved rewards. However, we can no longer put band-aids on a gaping wound. What's required is an overhaul of the way we settle cases and award damages, a new system that is completely outside of the conventional civil litigation system. A lay jury simply cannot be expected to understand the subtleties of a malpractice case, and to determine whether a physician or other healthcare professional acted inappropriately. If a practitioner is proven to be a repeat offender, there must be a mechanism to remediate or to remove her from practice. By necessity, sweeping federal legislation would be needed to achieve such a lofty goal. As with so many issues in our society, there are special interest groups, in this case trial attorneys, who will do whatever is necessary to preserve the flawed status quo if their income is at stake. And that includes aggressive lobbying of and copious donations to legislators in amounts that cannot be matched by medical professionals who have a lesser understanding of how to play the influence game.

PATIENT ADVICE
Where does this leave our patients? They must continue to advocate for tort reform and vote for legislators who are willing to aggressively pursue curative legislation. Only in this way will it be possible to lessen the burden on healthcare providers, understanding that care rendered by right-minded doctors and nurses will necessarily be superior to and safer than the flawed care that wounded and defensive practitioners will necessarily deliver.

If you believe you have been injured by the negligence of a healthcare provider, it is perfectly reasonable to ask questions of the caregivers with the hope of getting honest answers and a sincere apology. The offending parties may be willing to quickly provide compensation for the damages caused to avert a full-blown lawsuit. Having an attorney review the case should be your last resort and you will need to do whatever you can to find a reputable firm. Don't be afraid to be critical of legal opinion and to ask tough questions about litigation strategy. Remember that entering malpractice litigation can be psychologically damaging as old memories are resurrected and professional careers are placed in the balance, and that no matter how much money you or your family is awarded, the trauma of botched medical care will never be erased.

Story 4: The Rise of the Administrators

Scientists have announced the discovery of a new element called Administratium. This new element has no protons or electrons, thus having an atomic number of zero. It does, however, have 1 neutron, 125 assistant neutrons, 75 vice neutrons, and 111 assistant vice neutrons, giving it an atomic mass of 312. These 312 particles are held together by a force that involves the continuous exchange of meson-like particles called morons. (Adapted from Administratium: A 20th Anniversary Update by William DeBuvitz in Phys. Teach 2009; 47:33)

NARRATIVE

Mrs. Lopez was a 75-year-old Latina, in the hospital recovering from a somewhat difficult hysterectomy. During a routine examination, she was discovered to have uterine cancer that fortunately had been found early in its course, without evidence of spread. The surgery was supposed to be "minimally invasive," but halfway through the procedure, when the surgeon identified a couple of bleeding vessels, he decided to remove the uterus with an abdominal incision rather than extracting it through the vagina. Thus, Mrs. Lopez woke up with a large bandage on her abdomen and would have a scar she hadn't expected. She vaguely remembered someone telling her that an abdominal approach might be required but it hadn't completely registered with her. She had a great deal of incisional pain that she had been able to relieve with an intravenous morphine pump, but it had suddenly stopped working.

The pump began an incessant beeping, indicating that it had shut down just as Mrs. Lopez was having some of her worst post-operative pain. Unfortunately, she was alone. Her husband had been spending hours at her bedside, but he had gone out for lunch and wasn't due back for another hour.

Mrs. Lopez reached over and pushed the call button. No response, so she pushed it again and at least four more times over the next twenty minutes before a nurses' aide (who referred to herself as a "patient care technician") finally came to her bedside. Mrs. Lopez explained the situation. The technician confessed that he was not qualified to manipulate the morphine pump and would have to find a nurse to assist him. Another fifteen minutes went by before an obviously busy and harried nurse came in and with a few deft maneuvers, unclogged the intravenous line. The narcotic once again flowed into Mrs. Lopez's vein, to her decided relief.

But the story didn't end there. For the next three days of Mrs. Lopez's hospitalization, she continued to have issues with nursing care. She experienced long delays trying to get assistance, and the staff that did respond frequently couldn't address her problem definitively. Even simple chores like dressing changes took longer than expected, unappetizing meals arrived late and cold, and transport to imaging tests was unreliable. On one occasion, Mrs. Lopez was left stranded on a stretcher in a corridor in the radiology department for two hours and was rescued only because her husband went looking for her. Housekeeping was spotty. Her bathroom wasn't cleaned every day and not thoroughly when it was. Towels and linens arrived late in the day, if at all. Mrs. Lopez tired of being awakened every day by a phlebotomy technician. She couldn't understand why she needed so many blood tests and why the staff insisted on sticking a needle in her arm at 5:00 am. Sleep was hard enough without foolish interruptions.

Worse of all, the staff was just plain unhappy about their jobs, and that attitude spilled over into the way they related to the patients: always civil, rarely friendly, and never upbeat.

After three agonizing post-operative days, Mrs. Lopez was told that she had recovered sufficiently to be discharged. She and her husband were concerned because she had been out of bed only a few times and hadn't been able to use the bathroom alone. No matter, she was told that the hospital was crowded, and her discharge was overdue. If she stayed longer, it was likely that her insurance company wouldn't pay for the extra days and might even refuse coverage of her entire admission.

Leaving the hospital was another process that took several hours, as Mrs. Lopez waited for her paperwork, and then for the hospital's transportation services to bring a wheelchair to take her to the hospital entrance. But the coup de grace for Mrs. Lopez and her husband was the last-minute arrival of a woman in a long white lab coat, blocking the doorway, holding a clipboard. She explained she was a "patient experience specialist" from the

Quality Assurance Department who wanted to make sure that all had gone well during Mrs. Lopez's hospitalization. Anxious to be on their way, Mr. and Mrs. Lopez reassured the clueless clerk that everything had been just dandy, figuring that negative comments would only prompt more questions and cause a further delay in their escape from the hospital from hell.

Mrs. Lopez's recuperation at home took several weeks, and it was only because of her attentive husband that she was able to walk without pain. Her wound eventually healed, and she received good news at her postoperative visit: the tumor was confined to the uterus without evidence of spread. No further treatment would be necessary.

Over the next month, Mrs. Lopez was pilloried with emails and snail mail from the hospital, asking her to evaluate her hospital and surgical experience. She was so happy to be cancer-free, that she decided not to unload her frustrations with her hospital care, and simply deleted or trashed the inquiries before her husband, already angry about the six-figure hospital bill, could see the surveys and respond to them.

CASE EXPLANATION

Mrs. Lopez survived her hospitalization and eventually returned to normal function. Her care was in no way negligent or sub-standard. Her caregivers executed their tasks well enough for her to be discharged to her home, where she completed her recuperation, supervised by her husband. What was deficient was the *quality* of her hospital care and the many times she suffered needlessly physically as well as emotionally. And the reason for her discomfort was clear: there were not enough personnel to ensure that all her needs were adequately and promptly attended to.

As we will discuss in another vignette, hospitals are financially strapped for several reasons. Certainly, a reduction in fees and an increase in costs are the root cause. However, it is maddening that hospital leaders have chosen to spend money foolishly on administrative salaries, worthless marketing, failed initiatives, and ancillary services that bring little value to the routine care of hospitalized patients. There simply aren't enough nurses, patient care technicians, housekeepers, maintenance personnel, cafeteria staff, laboratory personnel, or patient transporters, and these shortages are especially acute during the evening and night shifts when patients are alone and most vulnerable. This situation has been referred to as "shrinkflation" or trying to do more work with fewer human resources.

Mrs. Lopez, like many patients, chose not to provide negative feedback about her hospitalization. Patients usually rate their care as being at least satisfactory even when conditions are clearly sub-standard. And even when a negative message is delivered, it is relatively easy for it to be excused away, never reaching any of those who are charged with maintaining quality of care. Until care deficiencies are addressed, erosion in quality will continue. Mistakes, in many cases lethal, plague modern medicine, and there is no evidence they are going away.

COMMENTARY

Hospitals across the United States are in financial trouble with narrow operating margins that in many cases have been firmly in the red. There is a myriad of reasons for this terrible development. The COVID-19 pandemic essentially shut down various medical and surgical services that make money for the hospitals, and while the aid they received from the government was helpful, it wasn't enough to make up for the accumulated deficits when the pandemic eased up. The costs of equipment and supplies, like everything else in an inflationary economy, increased dramatically and are not expected to recover any time soon. In essence, the cost of doing business for healthcare institutions has become prohibitive, causing the collapse and closure of rural as well as inner city hospitals. Those surviving have had to absorb the costs of caring for uninsured and under-insured patients who visit their emergency rooms with diseases out of control because of the dearth of primary care practices in their communities that could counsel prevention.

The assumption of care for indigent patients is not news. It is an expected part of the mission of nonprofit hospitals that preserve their tax-exempt status by rendering what is essentially charity care. What has changed is that insurance companies, led by Medicare, have ratcheted down their payments for a variety of medical services. Furthermore, those procedures that have been the gain leaders over the years have left the hospital entirely and migrated to surgical centers frequently owned by doctors and investors. As we will see in other stories, cataract surgery, colonoscopies, and joint replacement surgeries that used to keep the hospital in the black are now done elsewhere, leaving the hospitals with high-end surgical and intensive care for much sicker patients where the opportunity to make money is much lower.

The most blatantly absurd and egregious development has been the explosive growth in the number of healthcare administrators. But before we address the suits, it is important to understand how we got to this point.

The practice of medicine evolved slowly though the first three-quarters of the twentieth century. The traditional model was the solo practitioner who worked out of his (they were almost all men) office most of the time, but also rounded in the hospital to see and manage his patients there. With the increase in time and effort required to care for an expanded patient population, and the increasing complexity of the work itself, solo practices gave way to partnerships and physician-owned single specialty or multi-specialty groups.

What caused the most serious upheaval was the change in the business model. Whereas most medical care had been paid for out of pocket, rising sophistication meant higher costs that required insurance. Employers took on the responsibility of paying for health insurance for workers and their families as part of the "benefit package" commonly mandated in union contracts.

The game changer was Medicare, a government-funded system of care for older Americans. The entry of government into the medical care space had enormous ramifications because Congress, the executive branch, and even the judiciary, now had a reason to oversee and regulate medical care. This included setting payment for various services including doctor visits, laboratory tests, and medical and surgical procedures.

Dealing with Medicare, Medicaid and a growing assemblage of third-party payers became an enormous administrative task for physician-owned practices. An increasing percentage of the physician's time and attention had to be devoted to the business side of medicine. It wasn't long before people with business skills were incorporated into the medical office and hospital to assist with matters like billing, collection, scheduling, hiring and firing, facility planning, and numerous other chores that were required to keep the practice afloat.

Compounding the administrative load imposed by this changed business environment was government incursion into the practice of medicine itself. Legislators came to believe that they had the right to tell doctors and hospitals how to operate safely and effectively. Laws were passed at a dizzying rate that compelled doctors to report incidents, certify specific learnings, and care for patients in pre-defined ways. Many of these regulations have been associated not only with stiff fines for violations, but also the potential for criminal prosecution and imprisonment if ignored. As we will see in later stories, imposing all of this on doctors not only led to burn-out, but also accelerated the rate at which private practices gave up the ghost and allowed non-physician administrators to take over.

In most practices, doctors happily relinquished the administrative burden, although a few brave souls decided to embrace the challenge, obtained business degrees, and devoted an increasing amount of their time to administrative tasks. But it rapidly became clear that it would be nearly impossible to practice medicine at a high level while managing the business.

At the same time, medicine revenue generation was growing. As medical technology developed and new medicines and procedures were developed, costs escalated as did the salaries of physicians. The federal government, through Medicare and Medicaid, added billions to the medical care system. None of this enrichment of medicine escaped the notice of the corporate world. It rapidly became clear to corporate America that getting involved in medical care was a way to make a lot of money.

So, it was the perfect storm. Physicians who were generating enormous revenues felt overwhelmed to the point of ceding control of their practices to nonphysician business types, i.e. administrators (aka the suits), and it was game on.

Administratium has a normal half-life of about three years, at which point, it does not decay, but instead undergoes reorganization in which assistant neutrons, vice-neutrons and assistant vice-neutrons exchange places. Some studies have shown that the atomic mass actually increases after each reorganization. (ibid)

The first major inroad made by the suits was in the hospitals. Despite being "nonprofit" and traditionally poorly managed, these institutions had immense untapped revenue potential. But rapidly advancing technology, a growing demand for services, and more government regulation made running hospitals ever more complicated. It didn't take long for hospital boards and physician leadership to realize that help was needed. In the beginning, administrators migrated to hospital work from less lucrative industries. But it wasn't long before young and eager business types were able to enroll in a growing number of university degree programs dedicated to training healthcare administrators. No one could have predicted the explosion in the number of administrators each institution felt necessary for proper functioning. In the case of Mrs. Lopez, remember the patient experience specialist who visited her before discharge? How ironic that Mrs. Lopez would have had a much better experience if that clerk's salary had been allocated to a nurse to help Mrs. Lopez with her pain medication or to help get her back on her feet or to give her a bath.

So detached are administrators from the patient experience that they can fail even the most basic tasks, such as arranging adequate parking at their facility. A patient who is going to visit her doctor is necessarily anxious. The last thing that person wants to see is a long line of cars trying to enter a parking ramp, a guarantee that she will be late for her appointment. Or consider the patient who has received bad news from a healthcare provider and is desperate to go home and be with a loved one. Before she can do that, she must pay for parking at a kiosk that also has a long line and a complex set of instructions. Simple measures to help the beleaguered patient are not put into place, not because the responsible administrator is stupid, but because taking care of patients was not in their university's hospital administration curriculum.

A similar phenomenon of administration creep happened on the practice side, too. The physicians trying to keep their practices viable grew tired of the business-related work, including managing the EMR inbox. Seeing patients all day and then attending two-hour business meeting in the evening was not attractive or sustainable. A few physicians morphed into full-time administrators, but most ceded control to practice managers. Here, the proliferation was not as intense, but the focus of the practices changed radically. The imperative handed down from the practice directors was revenue generation and profit above all else. Physicians were no longer judged by the quality of their care, but rather the quantity of money-generating tests and procedures.

Research at other laboratories indicates that administratium occurs naturally in the atmosphere. It tends to concentrate at certain points such as government agencies, universities and most of all, health systems. It can usually be found in the newest, best appointed and sumptuous buildings and office suites. (ibid)

It would only be a short time before the real corporate raiders entered the scene. We are now dealing with healthcare systems and private equity firms buying practices with the intention of making an even greater profit. The overwhelming majority of doctors in the US are indentured, wholly owned by entities that are quite happy to set volume and revenue targets and to impose penalties on those who don't meet expectations. The unit of currency is RVUs or relative value units, the "value" of each physician task. Doctors are paid bonuses based on the number of RVUs they generate. Whether the tests they order or the procedures they carry out are necessary or performed skillfully is not a part of the equation.

And the best way to make money in the fee-for-service world we live in is to incentivize healthcare providers to see as many patients and to perform as many procedures as possible. The people who run hospitals and practices are usually not physicians and have no understanding of the core business. And yet, they set policies, hire and fire healthcare providers, and make daily decisions about how hospitals and practices do business, usually without meaningful input from doctors. Without any personal experience, administrators set revenue goals for healthcare workers including doctors and nurses, already struggling to keep up with a heavy workload that inevitably includes on call time and the completion of a wide variety of compulsory tasks imposed by clueless regulatory agencies.

Nurses, in particular, have taken the brunt of the cost saving measures. Their salaries have always been absurdly low, and they have felt disrespected and exploited. But nurses will never let their patients down, so administrators know they can be counted on to do whatever is necessary for their patients no matter how much they are paid and what perks they are denied. An example is day care. Since most nurses have children, the availability of easily accessible and affordable day care is vital. Hospitals used to provide that service for all their employees but, to save money, most of these facilities have gone away. Veteran and skilled nurses should feel insulted when administrators reward them with breakfast and a trinket on their national days of "recognition." Such paltry rewards merely underscore the fact that the tail *is* wagging the dog.

Since it has no electrons, administratium is inert. However, it can be detected chemically since it impedes every reaction with which it comes into contact. According to scientists, a minute amount of administratium causes a reaction that would occur in less than a second to take more than four months to complete. (ibid)

As they insinuated themselves deeper into the fabric of healthcare system, newly minted administrators learned quickly how to stack hospital boards with people like themselves, friends working in law, finance, and industry, who happily endorsed the business decisions of the hospital CEO. This included the hiring of several levels of administrators to share their burden, and the awarding of outrageous salaries, manyfold higher than the physicians and nurses who do the work. While the number of physicians has grown modestly over the past three decades, administrator proliferation has been exponential.

What hurts the most about the current situation is recent data showing that those few hospitals still run by physicians have better outcomes and generally higher quality of care than those run by non-physicians. And yet the bean counters, when they retire or move on to other lucrative jobs, are lauded for their vision and hard work. Their portraits are displayed prominently in hospital lobbies while they are provided with severance packages akin to the GDP of a small country. And they are replaced by people who have the same orientation and goals.

A new term has recently been coined in news media: "administrative harm." It means that administrators through misguided decisions can wreak as much havoc on patients as negligent healthcare providers. Mistakes can include bad decisions like closing hospital beds, or failing to do things that are necessary for good patient care, such as hiring more staff, almost always in the name of saving money or adhering to ridiculous regulations. Sadly, administrators have never been held to task for their errors, but it appears that much harm is done by people still being paid more money than they deserve. An administrator in California saw little problem with accepting a $25 million final salary after the healthcare system he was responsible for had to close the doors of several regional hospitals. When analyzed as pay units, CEO salaries may range from $2000 to $7000 per hour. While the recognition of administrative harm may finally begin to restore sanity to hospital management by holding incompetent people accountable, how best to prevent administrative mistakes remains to be seen.

CONCLUSION

In December of 2023, the *Philadelphia Inquirer* carried two healthcare stories in opposing columns in its metropolitan section. In the first story, nurses in two busy community hospitals had voted to strike. Their principal issue was salary. They were able to make a strong case that they weren't being paid at a level commensurate with their effort and amount of responsibility. The strike would last only a few days. After all, healthcare workers, unlike their bosses, can always be counted on to place their suffering patients ahead of their self-interests. The nurses eventually did win a modest pay raise, still not even close to their real value.

Whether by accident or design, the story in the next column was about the person who had assumed the acting presidency of a large university. His former position was the chief executive officer of the university's health system. The story detailed his credentials and the university's joy that this able person was willing to take on a complicated new task. In the last paragraph of the story, almost as an afterthought, the annual compensation of this healthcare administrator was listed as several million dollars. Such a ridiculous compensation package is not at all atypical. CEOs of nonprofit healthcare systems nationally have similarly outrageous annual salaries.

This mix of stories shows how much healthcare has been affected and often harmed by the rise of administrators. An already flawed system was turned on its head, putting bean counters at the top of the pyramid, able to dole out compensation and consideration to the "doers," the corps of hard-working professionals who do the work and generate revenue. There appears to be no relief in sight. Increasing regulation and oversight will mandate an even larger core of "checkers," which will inflate overhead, leaving less money for the core business of patient care.

PATIENT ADVICE

The message to take from this story is that patients must thoroughly investigate the practice and hospital they plan to frequent. Quality measures are hard to find or validate, but it may be possible to find out how your physician is compensated and by whom, and how they are or aren't incentivized.

While a return to the "good old days" of accountable and understandable family practice is unrealistic, I encourage you to do your homework and don't be afraid to ask tough questions when deciding on a new healthcare provider. It is still possible to enter a fruitful therapeutic relationship with eyes wide open.

Hospitals are a more complicated matter. Sources that rate hospitals like *US News and World Report* tend to focus on academic reputation and spend much less time analyzing the quality of bedside care. Be aware that hospitals will advertise how good they are by using reports from agencies that are paid a fee by the hospital they are evaluating for their analysis and rankings. Patient testimony in television commercials is usually scripted, will always be complimentary, and will rarely be helpful. In the end, lean on your primary care doctor and your learned friends to help you find the excellent personal care that we all desire and deserve.

And if, in the middle of the night, an ambulance comes to your home and transports you to the nearest hospital…well good luck with that.

Story 5: The Electronic Medical Record: Boon or Bane?

"One has a greater sense of degradation after an interview with a doctor than from any human experience." —Alice James

NARRATIVE

Mrs. Francis was a 55-year-old Caucasian woman living in the suburbs with her husband. They had no children; their only daughter had died suddenly when she was in her early twenties of unknown cause. They lived a simple life but were happy with their lot.

Mrs. Francis went to see her primary care physician because of chest congestion and a nagging cough. The doctor ordered a chest X-ray that didn't show any serious lung pathology but was remarkable for "widening of the mediastinum," the structure in the middle of the chest that houses, among other things, the aorta, the great vessel that channels blood out of the heart and carries it to the rest of the body. The exact cause of this widening was revealed by a CAT scan. Mrs. Francis had a thoracic aortic aneurysm, a weakening in the wall of the aorta where it exits the heart. This is a serious situation because aneurysms can burst or tear and if they do, death is a likely outcome because of the fast rate at which blood under high pressure will leave the circulatory system and leak into the lungs and chest cavity. How likely an aneurysm is to burst, or shred, is determined by several factors. The most important is its size. The larger the aneurysm, the greater the chance of a catastrophic rupture.

Fortunately for Mrs. Francis, the aneurysm at its largest diameter was only four centimeters. Although there may be exceptions, five centimeters is the aortic root size that is ordinarily a cause for concern. The cardiologist to whom she was sent for a consultation told her that she was fine for the time being, but she would require yearly CAT scans to make sure that the aneurysm wasn't enlarging. If or when it did, surgery might be required to remove the weakened segment of the aorta and replace it with a plastic graft. The doctor reassured her that her heart muscle was functioning well and wasn't dilated. Most of her aorta, including the aortic valve, which sits at the point where the aorta leaves the heart's pumping chamber, looked normal. She was told that the surgery would be straightforward and could be accomplished with "acceptable risk" but only if it was performed at a center with experience doing that kind of operation.

Mrs. Francis was relieved to hear that her situation was stable and agreed to have routine follow-up appointments. She also understood that if she ever had chest pain or intense shortness of breath, or felt like she was going to pass out, she would need to go to an emergency room as quickly as possible.

For the next five years, Mrs. Francis visited the cardiologist annually. At each visit, he performed an echocardiogram to make sure her valves were functioning normally, and her heart was not enlarged, and then ordered a CAT scan to measure aortic size. Every year, Mrs. Francis anxiously awaited the phone call from the doctor's office to let her know whether her aneurysm had grown, and each year she was grateful to learn that it was stable. She had no symptoms and was able to go about all her activities including walking with her husband on a regular basis, which she enjoyed greatly.

It so happened that, besides a comfortable residence in the suburbs, Mrs. Francis and her husband had a small vacation home not far away in the mountains that they visited mostly on weekends. While sitting in front of a fire one winter Saturday evening, Mrs. Francis had the sudden onset of a sharp pain in the middle of her chest, so severe that it literally took her breath away. When the pain continued, her husband called 911. Mrs. Francis lay on the sofa, comforted by her husband, trying desperately to hold on to her senses. By the time the ambulance arrived, Mrs. Francis's pain had mostly subsided, but the EMTs advised that a visit to the hospital would be a good idea.

On arrival, Mrs. Francis was greeted by a friendly triage nurse who took her medical history. Mrs. Francis related that she had a diagnosis of an "aortic aneurysm" that was being imaged on a regular basis and was stable. The nurse, however, mistakenly recorded that Mrs. Francis had an *abdominal* aneurysm, a more common entity than a thoracic aneurysm. An abdominal aneurysm is a weakness of the aortic wall as the aorta travels through the abdomen, supplying blood to the stomach, liver and kidneys. In other words, the abdominal aorta is housed in a totally different part of the body than the thoracic aorta. This incorrect notation was placed in the electronic medical record (EMR), as well as cut and pasted into every subsequent healthcare provider's note during Mrs. Francis's two-day hospitalization.

Since no one had established that Mrs. Francis had an aneurysm in her chest, the pain she suffered was assumed to have come from the lungs or maybe the heart itself. Therefore, the testing she had in the hospital was to rule out a clot in the lungs or a coronary artery blockage. She had a chest X-ray that showed a widened mediastinum, but it was mistakenly read as normal by a moonlighting radiologist whom the hospital had hired for weekend coverage, even though he wasn't board-certified.

Mrs. Francis's other tests came back mostly normal except for a mildly elevated level of cardiac troponin, a cardiac enzyme that, when elevated, indicates heart damage; this finding was regarded as a possible explanation of her chest pain. Based on that result, the ER doctor decided to have her admitted for more blood tests. He was not going to assume the liability for discharging a chest pain patient he didn't know. To his credit, while filling out her admitting history and physical examination, he tried to go online to obtain records from Mrs. Francis's caregivers in the city. Because the facilities where she had her CAT scans done had a different EMR vendor than at his hospital, accessing the records electronically was impossible. His search was fruitless.

In the hospital, the fiasco continued. When the hospital doctor who was assigned to Mrs. Francis's case saw the triage nurse's note about an aortic abdominal aneurysm, he ordered an abdominal ultrasound to make sure it was not enlarged or ruptured. He doubted the chest pain was caused by an abdominal aneurysm, but he wanted to be thorough. He was happy to get a report back only a few hours later saying that the abdominal aorta was "ectatic" (crooked) but of relatively normal size. He made a note of it in the EMR but forgot to relay the information to the patient, who had been confused by the need to have a test of her abdomen. Mrs. Francis didn't ask the person doing the test or any of the nurses why it was ordered in the first place.

When all the hospital tests came back as normal, and when Mrs. Francis felt better, she was discharged and told to follow-up with her primary care doctor. Since it was a Sunday, no one called her private doctor or transmitted any of the hospital information to that physician's office. They needn't have bothered. The primary care doctor had never installed an EMR system in her office because of the expense. She relied instead on fax, phone and snail mail to get and send information about her patients. If the doctor ever wanted to know what happened to Mrs. Francis at the hospital in the mountains, she would have had to fax a request signed by the patient to that hospital's medical records department.

None of this lack of communication made much of a difference because only a few hours after Mrs. Francis arrived back to her primary home, she had another severe bout of chest pain. She was brought to the local ER where a CAT scan of her chest revealed that the aneurysm had dissected, meaning that her aorta had shredded, with blood leaking into the wall of the vessel and into adjacent structures in her chest.

The situation was grave. Mrs. Francis was taken directly from the ER to the operating room. The heart surgeon who was covering emergencies had little experience with repairing aortic aneurysms but that also didn't make a difference. Mrs. Francis had no chance of surviving the catastrophic dissection and was declared dead on the OR table an hour later.

CASE EXPLANATION

This sad case has several important learning points, but let's make sure the facts are clear. Mrs. Francis had a *thoracic* aortic aneurysm. Why? There are several possible reasons, including a hereditary disease called Marfan's syndrome, associated with, among other things, tall stature and long fingers and toes, which Mrs. Francis didn't have. She also had no known family history of a similar condition, and had never been a smoker, both strong risk factors for aortic disease. But Mrs. Francis may have had a familial predisposition to this sort of aneurysm, and her daughter's premature death may have been a clue. Since there was no autopsy, we don't know if her daughter died suddenly of a ruptured aorta. Unfortunately, her cardiologist didn't take a complete family history and didn't order genetic testing. He assumed that, as in most cases, hers was simply a sporadic case for which a cause would never be identified. This was also a mistake because Mrs. Francis's genetic testing results may have been useful for counseling and screening members of her family.

Another alarming aspect of this case is the failure of the surveillance plan put in place for Mrs. Francis to prevent the catastrophe. Over five years, her aneurysm had not grown significantly but, without warning, it dissected. Medicine is a science of probability and not certainty. For most patients with thoracic aneurysms, surveillance does work to delay surgery with its attendant risks until it is necessary, and this is important for several reasons. Despite what the cardiologist said about "acceptable risk," replacement of the thoracic aorta is serious business since it may also require aortic valve replacement and reattachment of the coronary arteries where they exit the aorta to supply the heart muscle. In addition, artificial grafts don't last forever. The longer one can forestall surgery, the better the chances of needing the surgery only once. Finally, technology moves quickly, and the development of better treatment methods, such as repair through catheters without the need for surgery, might be possible as years go by.

But in a small percentage of patients, despite best intentions and compliance with regular testing, a calamity happens. The tragedy of Mrs. Francis's case is that there was a warning. The Saturday night episode of chest pain probably represented a small tear in the vessel that, by some miracle, didn't extend until the following Monday, after she had been discharged from the hospital.

Could Mrs. Francis have been saved if the dissection had been diagnosed in the emergency room the Saturday before her death? We can't know for sure. Much would have depended on how quickly she would have been referred to a center with sufficient expertise to do the operation, and the skill of the surgeon. However, there is no question that her *probability* of survival would have been much higher if the operation had started when she was stable and in relatively good condition. Instead, without accurate information and the inability to obtain Mrs. Francis' records, the ER staff went about their business of ordering irrelevant tests as recommended in the "chest pain template" in their EMR, and then depending on misleading results to rationalize discharge after a fruitless admission to the hospital. When the tear extended, Mrs. Francis had virtually no chance of survival.

COMMENTARY

There are several issues regarding medical record keeping, which is the focus of this case. First, we recognize that the medical record is a sacred document. It is supposed to contain all the relevant medical information about a patient. There must be easy access for practitioners with utterly clear and decipherable information. As we have seen, the very lives of patients depend on medical record accuracy.

Because of the importance of the medical record, maintaining it properly is a burden on doctors and other healthcare providers that is seriously underestimated. To document all elements of patient care is an onerous task. It has been made even more unpalatable with the advent of the EMR. Though it may have some advantages for patient care, transition from paper to an electronic record was mandated by hospitals and insurers for one principal reason: to secure payment. For doctors and hospitals to be reimbursed for their work by third parties, the medical record must contain proof that healthcare providers obtained relevant historical information, examined the patient and ordered and reviewed indicated laboratory tests before prescribing medication or carrying out procedures. Several items need to be included in every visit including diagnostic codes linked to orders for medications and laboratory studies. Using templates, administrators can be more confident that payment will be made efficiently and promptly by insurers.

EMR maintenance is a time-consuming task, and so shortcuts are frequently employed. One of these is the "cut and paste" tactic used in Mrs. Francis's case. Instead of the second and third person who saw Mrs. Francis asking her about her history and entering what they learned, each of them complied with the need for "documentation" by simply copying what was already in the chart, which in this case was literally dead wrong. Mrs. Francis had an aneurysm in her chest, not her abdomen. A falsehood was perpetuated and ultimately Mrs. Francis, who didn't have the medical sophistication to put the doctor and nurses right, paid a dear price. My fourth Philip Sarkis mystery novel, *Death on the Pole*, includes a similar story in which failure to report the details of a woman's resuscitation out of the hospital led to an inaccurate diagnosis of a congenital arrhythmia syndrome that resulted in inadequate management, an avoidable death, a nasty lawsuit, and of course, grisly murders to follow.

Another short-cut used ubiquitously in the EMR is the generic template, a set of passages of various length that summarize a fact or finding that is so common that it can be pasted in its entirety into a patient note. However, no two patients are ever the same, so unless the EMR writer (e.g. the doctor or nurse) edits the template carefully, it's highly probable that some of this generic template information will be irrelevant at best, or at the worst, just plain wrong. An example is a template of a normal physical examination that is used by residents and interns in lieu of typing in all the details for each of the many hospital admissions they are expected to oversee. If the patient has an abnormality or two, the EMR writer must change the template, but that step is frequently forgotten. What emerges is the absurdity of a patient admitted with severe heart valve disease when the EMR says that on physical examination "heart sounds were normal and there were no murmurs."

Another consequence of the introduction of the EMR has been a deterioration in the quality of physician communication. During my fellowship training I was taught that the letter I sent as a consultant to the referring physician was a critically important document. It needed to briefly summarize the patient's situation and examination, list all the relevant facts about diagnostic tests and treatments, and deliver a succinct and well thought out summary with precise recommendations. All of this should be contained in a letter of no more than two pages because anything more than that wouldn't be read or absorbed by a busy clinician.

Shortly after the EMR came online, I noticed that the cogent consultant letters I used to receive or read in the medical record were replaced by ten to twenty-page documents. These "letters" contained just about every conceivable detail about the patient including remote laboratory and imaging test results and previous notes that had no relevance to the current situation. There was a bewildering repetition of known facts that made no sense in the context of the present illness, retained simply because the writer didn't have the time to omit or edit them.

Why did all of this happen? Because hospital administrators decided that dictating letters was too expensive and that doctors and nurses could do it themselves using templates and "cut and paste" shortcuts to avoid spending the time required to write a better letter or the money required to pay a transcription service. I stubbornly continued to dictate my letters and was frequently told by my referring physicians how informational my two-page letters were and how easy they were to read.

As for the letters I received, I was faced with two choices. I could try to speed-read the tomes, or I could ignore most of the content and scroll through, searching for the most important part, the clinical impression and plan. I did either or both depending on the circumstances, muttering obscenities as I read through the verbiage. What saves time for one person adds frustration to someone further down the line. To say nothing of the possibility of missing important data.

Because of repetitive information, the EMR on complicated patients can grow to ludicrous lengths. I was recently asked to review records in a case in which a patient died after having a major seizure. I was asked if there was any possibility that the victim had occult cardiac disease that may have contributed to her death. When I opened the hospital records, I found nearly three thousand pages of information regarding a six-day hospitalization. I spent hours combing through reams of extraneous and repetitive information to find a few pages or relevant data.

Mention the word *inbox* to most doctors and they cringe. From a variety of sources, messages, lab reports, patient calls, orders to be signed, and just about anything else that goes into patient care gets dumped into the physician's EMR inbox. Many doctors, especially obsessive-compulsive types like me, check their inbox several times a day, attempting, without success, to keep it empty or nearly so. Others ignore it and let the number of items grow to an absurd number before they finally give in and spend hours trying to untangle the mess. This latter is a dangerous practice because especially important messages will be buried in the avalanche of "for your information" notes that accumulate hourly.

It is important for patients to understand that inbox management is an add-on to all the other things doctors are expected to do with their day. Inbox work is not reimbursed by most payers, and while we manage the inbox, we have less time to talk to patients on the phone or in person.

The EMR inbox has also pretty much guaranteed that there are no more doctor days off. If a physician wants to take excellent care of his or her patients, messages must be checked. Deferring to an overworked covering partner to answer your queries doesn't work well because that person doesn't know your patient, and that person's responses are likely to be incomplete or unsatisfactory. Better to take an hour in the middle of a weekend day or holiday to "check the inbox," to remain apprised of developments and to intervene if necessary. The alternative is to return from vacation to face a series of calamities and misunderstandings.

The proponents of the EMR have long been attracted to what has been referred to as "interoperability," or the ability to access medical records from another healthcare facility. And the truth is that such access is possible and used regularly. However, EMRs have never been standardized, and several different systems still exist. At the beginning of computerization of medical records, the government unwisely decided to let the market decide which EMRs would emerge as the favorites. This, even though the Veterans Administration had already developed a perfectly good and user-friendly system that could have been sold and installed for a fraction of the cost that commercial firms have charged. And continue to charge, as they roll out expensive "upgrades" that almost never make work easier but wreak havoc for several weeks until all the users acclimate to the new features and screens.

Amazingly, there are still some holdouts who use old-fashioned do-it-yourself systems in their office or have no EMR at all, even though some payers refuse to reimburse healthcare providers who don't use computers. As we saw in Mrs. Francis' case, obtaining or sending records, especially in an emergency or during off-hours, can be difficult if not impossible, so hard in fact, that most healthcare providers don't even make the effort. In this case, not knowing that the aneurysm was in Mrs. Francis's chest and not in her belly had disastrous consequences.

Most healthcare providers were happy to have the EMR as we dove into telemedicine during the COVID pandemic. It provided a way to facilitate communication with our patients, especially those who were tech-savvy enough to do video visits. But legislators and payers have not supported the continuation of telemedicine in the post-pandemic world, either because of inter-state licensing restrictions or because of payer reluctance to reimburse for more frequent patient visits. They continue to pay only for visits that have a "video component" even though most elderly patients can use a phone but not Zoom. For this and other reasons, telemedicine, one of the few things the EMR was good for, now withers on the vine.

There are several opportunities for improvement, but most have not been implemented rapidly or extensively. For example, one obvious fix is the use of scribes, people with a modicum of medical training who can sit at the computer during a patient encounter and enter all the relevant patient information while the physician talks to and examines the patient. The scribe also generates a summary of the visit, edited by the physician with a personal cover note to the referring doctor, outlining the essential facts and recommendations. Scribes cost money but the number of patients who could be seen by a practitioner is multiplied and their use more than pays for the service. Think about how much faster you might be able to get an appointment with a consultant if throughput were accelerated, not to mention removing an enormous burden from the physician.

Several privately owned physician practices have seen the light and employ scribes, but most practices owned by healthcare systems have not, insisting that the expense is not warranted. They would have a point if employed physicians work as indentured servants rather than professional healers. As you will see when I discuss hospital administrators, it is just this kind of rational and effective solution that they reject out of hand. Without a working knowledge of what the clinician is encountering daily, administrators remain resistant to measures that would clearly improve the quality of patient care. My latest plea to an administrator about scribes was countered by the statement that we would soon have artificial intelligence to help us in the office. When and how that will happen, and how much that intervention will cost weren't included in his desultory reply.

CONCLUSION

The transition to an electronic medical record was inevitable. Many thought that physician resistance to transitioning to electronic records was short-sighted and downright stupid, and it may have been. On the other hand, doctors knew that imposing such a large burden would necessarily lead to a deterioration of care. They eventually capitulated, but it turns out the doctors were correct.

What has emerged is a doctor-eating monster that jeopardizes medical care, distracts physicians from patients who are eager for their attention, interrupts a doctor's family life, and consumes her or his free time. No one could have anticipated the upheaval that the EMR has visited on doctors and patients. The roll-out was chaotic, with multiple vendors vying for vast business opportunities, in many cases selling EMR systems that were poorly conceived and doomed to failure. There was also a fundamental under-appreciation of how computer unsavvy doctors are, and so the learning curves were steep, especially for the large percentage of practicing doctors over the age of 55 or 60. I had terribly competent senior colleagues who left the profession solely because they didn't want to spend an enormous amount of time and energy learning how to use an EMR, especially with only a few years left in practice.

We are left with an imperfect system with little hope for rapid or substantial improvement. The entry of younger and more tech-savvy doctors and pressure from patients and payers to improve the situation may help over the long haul. Yet, we should not expect better expertise, or that the implementation of artificial intelligence will solve the fundamental issue of practitioner disconnection from patients; in fact, the latter will likely make things worse. Expensive litigation resulting from fixable imperfections may one day effect meaningful change, including hiring medical scribes for all practitioners. But for now, clinicians and their patients suffer quietly.

PATIENT ADVICE

Patient access to medical records is one of the benefits that the EMR makes possible. However, patients aren't always able to interpret test results themselves and become frightened by terminology that sounds ominous. Going over all your reports with your healthcare provider is essential so that you can understand them. In any healthcare situation, like the emergency room, it is optimal to make a new provider aware of accessibility to your records and what they may contain. Information that is relevant to your current illness will facilitate your care and reduce the chances of unnecessary testing or missed diagnoses. Interoperability, that is the ability of one EMR system to communicate with another, is becoming more commonplace, and is worthy of discussion with your physician and local healthcare system. Delivery of seamless care can be used as a priority in selecting where you would like to have your medical care delivered and by whom.

It is also reasonable to search for practices that use medical scribes with the expectation that you will spend more quality time with the doctor in the office. Insisting that your doctor talk to you instead of facing a computer screen and typing away is not unreasonable. Don't let the EMR get in the way of quality healthcare.

Story 6: Precertification Doesn't "Certify" Anything

"I got the bill for my surgey. Now I know why those doctors were wearing masks." —James H. Boren

NARRATIVE

Mrs. Dowd was an active 70-year-old Caucasian woman in good health. She exercised regularly and tried to pursue a good diet. She and her husband were "foodies" who bought only organic foods, frequently cooked in, and tried to maintain a balanced diet. Her primary care doctor was satisfied with her blood pressure control using an ACE-inhibitor, and she also took metformin for early diabetes. Her cholesterol was a bit high, but she had severe muscle cramps with a statin and didn't want to pay a large price for one of the new alternative drugs. All of these "risk factors" were particularly important in Mrs. Dowd's case because several people in her family had coronary artery disease, including her mother, who died of a heart attack at the age of 60 and two sisters who required cardiac catheterization and stent placement. Granted, most of the women in her family who had a coronary problem were smokers, but Mrs. Dowd was taking no chances, and neither was her primary care doctor. When Mrs. Dowd herself developed chest pain, it wasn't ignored.

One nice day, while walking her dog in her neighborhood, Mrs. Dowd experienced a burning sensation in the middle of her chest that didn't radiate but was accompanied by a touch of breathlessness and nausea. The discomfort lasted only a minute or two and she was able to return home. She immediately called her doctor, who recommended a visit the next day, and rest at home in the meantime.

At that visit, Mrs. Dowd's examination and electrocardiogram were normal, and subsequent lab tests were not concerning. Given her description of her symptoms, her doctor thought that she might have had reflux, but given her family history, he recommended a cardiology consultation, which he arranged for her to have within a few days.

The cardiologist who saw her, Dr. Thom, was concerned. She offered several options to Mrs. Dowd including a CAT scan, catheterization, or a stress test. Dr. Thom favored the last option since it would provide a good deal of information about her heart structure and function and exclude the presence of significant coronary artery disease with minimal risk and no radiation exposure. Mrs. Dowd agreed and so an exercise-echocardiogram, done with electrocardiogram and ultrasound imaging, was scheduled for later in the week at Dr. Thom's office.

This is when the ordeal started. Mrs. Dowd had a Medicare Advantage plan. As we saw in a previous story, the insurance company that managed her healthcare plan had become convinced that doctors were ordering too many stress tests with heart imaging. They therefore mandated a review before exercise-echocardiograms would be paid for. Dr. Thom's office anticipated the company's response and submitted the appropriate documentation, but learned the next day that the test was denied. In an email, the company said that an exercise-echocardiogram was not indicated, and that Mrs. Dowd should have a "regular" exercise test. She would be permitted to walk on a treadmill while her electrocardiogram was monitored, but they didn't think she needed direct imaging of her heart with ultrasound to determine if it was getting adequate blood flow through the coronary arteries.

Dr. Thom was not surprised. She had been through this process several times with many insurance companies. Her first response was to send a dissenting email, hoping that the company would concede that carrying out a regular exercise test was inadequate. It is well established that the electrocardiogram is not as useful in women as in men; there is a high false positive rate, which means the test may indicate a problem when none exists. Dr. Thom also wanted information about Mrs. Dowd's cardiac function, information easily accrued with ultrasound and not with an electrocardiogram alone.

Despite several subsequent emails and phone calls, the insurance company wouldn't budge. Dr. Thom had the office call Mrs. Dowd to see if she wanted to pay for the test herself. The full price of the test, without the usual insurance company discount, was $5,000. Mrs. Dowd's response was expected: no, thank you. So, after discussing the situation, Dr. Thom and Mrs. Dowd agreed to give in to the insurance company and proceed with a simple exercise test.

The test went well. Mrs. Dowd had an excellent exercise capacity with an appropriate rise in heart rate and blood pressure, and she had a normal heart rhythm throughout the test. She had a twinge of chest discomfort at peak exercise, but the problem was that her electrocardiogram was distinctly abnormal. Her ST segments, or the portion of the tracing that reflected the adequacy of her coronary circulation, dropped one millimeter, a result that suggested a blockage in one or more of her coronary arteries.

Dr. Thom, who supervised the test, told Mrs. Dowd and her husband that she didn't know if the result was a true or false positive. They again discussed alternatives including a CAT scan to look directly at the coronary arteries, a cardiac catheterization to squirt dye into the arteries and then view them on x-ray, or another stress test, this time with nuclear imaging to determine if the heart muscle was getting enough blood. Mrs. Dowd's sister had had a bad experience with her catheterization, and Mrs. Dowd was afraid of the large radiation exposure from the CAT scan, so she favored a nuclear stress test that carried minimal radiation risk. That test wasn't available at Dr. Thom's office. It would need to be carried out at the local hospital's laboratory, which would take a week or two to schedule. Dr. Thom didn't think the delay would be a problem if Mrs. Dowd did not overexert.

This time, considering Mrs. Dowd's abnormal stress test result, the insurance company approved the nuclear study. However, three days before the test, Mrs. Dowd, while preparing breakfast for her husband, developed the same burning in her chest, but now it was much more severe. Her husband called 911 but before the ambulance arrived, Mrs. Dowd collapsed. Her husband tried to perform CPR but had never been properly trained. The ambulance arrived ten minutes later and was able to defibrillate Mrs. Dowd's heart into a normal rhythm and her blood pressure rapidly recovered as well. She was transported to the hospital, where she was intubated. Her electrocardiogram now indicated she had at least one closed coronary artery, the circumflex coronary artery, the occlusion of which is sometimes difficult to detect by the electrocardiogram alone. She was taken to the catheterization laboratory where the vessel supplying blood to the side and bottom of her heart was relieved of a significant stenosis and a stent was placed.

Mrs. Dowd received excellent post-resuscitative care in the hospital including cooling of her body in the ICU in the hopes of preserving as much of her brain function as possible. Almost all her organs, including her heart, recovered well but the prolonged period of cardiac arrest had partially damaged her brain. Though she was able to go home after a lengthy stay at a rehabilitation facility, she had permanent memory and speech impairments that significantly reduced her quality of life.

CASE EXPLANATION

As her primary care doctor and Dr. Thom had feared, Mrs. Dowd had coronary artery disease. The chest burning she experienced when she was walking her dog was angina pectoris, or pain caused when the heart muscle is deprived of sufficient blood flow and oxygenation. As so often happens in women, the discomfort was not "typical." That is, she didn't suffer a squeezing sensation, the pain didn't radiate into her jaw or left arm, and she didn't break out into a sweat.

Why women have a somewhat different set of symptoms isn't completely understood but cardiologists have learned to take seriously any chest, back or even abdominal discomfort in women, especially those like Mrs. Dowd who have a positive family history. Most compelling was that Mrs. Dowd had several relatively young women in her family with significant coronary artery disease. This fact, along with her high blood pressure and early diabetes, placed her at a relatively high risk of vascular disease.

Fortunately, Dr. Thom reacted to Mrs. Dowd's complaints appropriately and offered her a variety of options to determine if she had a severe coronary problem. Using what has been referred to as "shared decision making," they decided to go forward with an exercise echocardiogram. This is a commonly ordered test in cardiology practice because, as Dr. Thom explained, it has good predictive accuracy, and it provides comprehensive information that would be helpful in managing Mrs. Dowd's coronary artery disease. For example, knowing if her heart function was normal or abnormal would not only have a powerful impact on her prognosis, but it would also heavily impact the choice of drugs or interventions to treat her. The test is easy on the patient, without the need for an intravenous line or drug injections. It is also relatively fast, taking about a half hour to complete in most centers.

Unfortunately, the exercise-echocardiogram is overutilized by some practitioners who can easily set up a stress test facility in their office and use it even in low-risk individuals to maximize income. Therefore, exercise-echocardiography appears on the long list of diagnostic tests for which "pre-certification" is required. According to the insurance company's operation manual, Mrs. Dowd didn't have enough of a reason to have the test, and so, over Dr. Thom's objections, it was denied.

Dr. Thom advised Mrs. Dowd that she could have the exercise echocardiogram if she paid for it herself. Dr. Thom's practice was owned by a healthcare system that had a published price list for tests. In the case of an exercise echocardiogram, the retail price was $5,000, roughly five times what the insurance company would pay, and ten times the true cost of the test. Not surprisingly, Mrs. Dowd declined that option, so Dr. Thom went forward with a no-frills exercise test. The results suggested the presence of coronary artery disease but needed confirmation.

The other three options that were available to Mrs. Dowd at that point were all reasonable and would have been useful. Once again, Dr. Thom presented each to Mrs. Dowd, who made an informed decision to have another exercise test. Dr. Thom believed nuclear imaging during exercise stress would yield a reliable result. Radiation exposure, a concern of Mrs. Dowd, would be much less than with the CAT scan, and would carry much less hazard than a cardiac catheterization, another option that worried Mrs. Dowd.

What Dr. Thom did not emphasize with Mrs. Dowd and her husband was that during the several-day waiting period for the exercise nuclear test, there was a small risk that she could have another bout of chest discomfort, even without exertion. Unfortunately, knowing when a vulnerable plaque in the coronary artery will chose to become unstable and rupture to occlude the vessel is impossible. With an abundance of bad luck, Mrs. Dowd not only had a more severe coronary artery event, but this time the lack of blood flow to the heart muscle rendered it electrically unstable and she had a cardiac arrest. The resuscitation saved her life, but the brain, the most oxygen sensitive organ in the body, was damaged enough to keep her from resuming her normal active life.

When Mrs. Dowd did not recover normal function in the rehabilitation hospital, Mr. Dowd was made aware that his wife was going to need expensive care at a nursing facility. If they opted for home care, she would need a full-time caregiver. Since her heart and kidneys and other organs had recovered, her life expectancy, though shortened, could extend out several years. Mr. and Mrs. Dowd had a reasonable amount of money put aside for their retirement, but their medical insurance company, the same one that had precipitated the crisis by not approving the test Dr. Thom had recommended in the first place, made it clear that they would pay only a modest portion of the cost of day-to-day custodial care.

Mr. Dowd promptly consulted a malpractice firm, known to him because of its glitzy television advertisement, to determine if Mrs. Dowd's care had been negligent. A lawyer cousin had advised him to do so, on the premise that the stress nuclear study could have been performed sooner. Mr. Dowd was particularly interested in suing the medical insurance company that had denied the exercise-echocardiogram. The young attorney with whom he spoke explained that medical insurance companies cannot be sued for malpractice.

However, after a thorough review, the malpractice attorneys told Mr. Dowd that a case could be made that Dr. Thom had been negligent for not making it clear to Mrs. Dowd that a delay in getting her nuclear test placed her at risk. They had carefully examined Dr. Thom's notes and letters, and such a warning was not documented anywhere in the record. Mr. Dowd was reluctant to pursue a case against Dr. Thom, whom he perceived to be a kind and caring person, but he was told that if he wanted a financial award, he had no choice. So, Dr. Thom was sued for negligence in her handling of Mrs. Dowd's case.

Dr. Thom was devastated, convinced in her own mind that she had communicated effectively with Mr. and Mrs. Dowd, and that she had been victimized by a stubborn health insurer. Her first instinct was to fight hard to defend herself.

The initial phases of the case didn't go well for Dr. Thom. With the insurance company off the hook, it was clear that Dr. Thom and her healthcare system would have to absorb the total burden of a verdict against them. Even though Dr. Thom's office was in the suburbs of the city, the health system had offices in the city itself. Therefore, the lawsuit was brought in a municipal court where plaintiffs win more frequently, and the verdicts are much higher. Representing Mr. Dowd were plaintiff attorneys, famous for their toughness and success. They had identified two cardiologists who were listed as "Yale doctors." In reality, they practiced in a backwater hospital loosely affiliated with the university health system. Each was willing to testify in court that Dr. Thom had been recklessly negligent in not ordering a catheterization immediately, and that her decision to wait for the nuclear study was a substantial deviation from the standard of care. The plaintiff attorneys let it be known that they intended to seek punitive damages in the case, which were not covered by insurance. If awarded, the punitive damages would have to be paid by Dr. Thom personally.

Dr. Thom's defense attorneys were provided by her healthcare system, which was eager to settle the case and avoid the terrible publicity it would entail. Dr. Thom's opinion about her innocence was the last thing they were worried about. They knew that an alleged wrongful death in a malpractice case is an awful situation, but not nearly as bad as having a brain-damaged plaintiff drooling in front of a lay jury for several days while attorneys argued about who was responsible for her plight.

Ultimately, Dr. Thom gave in and agreed to a two-million-dollar settlement, to the limits of her malpractice insurance policy in exchange for being relieved of any punitive damages. For her, it was the final straw. She had been seriously considering leaving clinical practice and going to work for a pharmaceutical company, and now her decision was solidified. As we saw in our vignette about Mrs. Apple, a medical malpractice case has multiple victims. In this case, not only was a good-hearted, vital person's life wrecked, but a helpful and experienced doctor would be saying goodbye to her sad patients.

COMMENTARY

You might think that this case is an extreme example of what can happen when proper care is deferred. Rest assured that when patients at risk are not cared for properly and promptly, bad things happen. Some of the consequences may not be as dramatic as what occurred in Mrs. Dowd's case, but punctual, meticulous, thoughtful patient management always pays dividends for the patient and for the healthcare provider. Care deferred is frequently care denied.

Mrs. Dowd's case was devastating for her and her family. Almost every one of my patients, when asked if they would rather die or have a catastrophic stroke or brain damage, will chose the former. They cite not wanting to be a burden on their loved ones and suffering the indignity of custodial care. Brain damage, such as Mrs. Dowd suffered, is not treatable or reversible. In essence, she lost her humanity, and her husband lost his wife.

Besides the personal tragedy, Mrs. Dowd's case will impose a terrible cost on the healthcare system. The cost of caring for her for the remaining years of her life will easily reach seven and maybe eight figures. Who will bear that financial burden? To begin, it will be Medicare and her insurance carrier. Ironically, the company that attempted to limit the cost of care will end up spending orders of magnitude more money to support Mrs. Dowd in her home or wherever she is institutionalized. But as we learned, the insurers are careful to limit the amount of money and the length of time they will contribute to the care of a brain-damaged person. What happens when those payments end or are severely curtailed? The patient and her family become responsible for the costs and in most cases, their savings are depleted rapidly. They may choose to assume debt but there is no bottom to the well. Unpaid medical bills is the most frequent cause of bankruptcy for private citizens in the US.

Once the money is gone, the final step is institutionalization in a facility that is supported by public funds. These nursing homes are notorious for how poorly staffed and supplied they are, and how substandard the care of the residents can be. When one considers all these consequences, there can be no argument that the story of Mrs. Dowd is a tragedy of mind-blowing proportions. It was the fear of financial ruin, more than a need for retribution, that prompted Mr. Dowd to hire a malpractice firm and sue Dr. Thom.

But let us return to the fundamental lesson of this vignette: companies that finance healthcare, and are sanctioned to do so by your government, are permitted to countermand physician decisions about patient care, and to do so without recourse, including immunity from civil action. They are effectively protected by laws that limit their liability no matter how outrageous and reckless their decisions are.

Precisely how we arrived at this ridiculous place in patient care is difficult to discern. Clearly, when health insurance was first conceived about a century ago, there was no intention of getting in the way of good medical care. But several things have happened over the last fifty years that corrupted the system. First, though regulated, there has been no attempt to stop medical insurance companies from making substantial profits, much of which is deposited in offshore accounts. Their "non-profit" designation is a misnomer, allowing them to pay little or no tax while continuing to compensate their executives with lavish salaries while working in luxurious office buildings.

The rationale used by insurance companies for the copious capital accumulation is that they need reserve funds for contingencies like a global pandemic. The flaw in that argument is that medical insurance companies are not susceptible to fund depletion from a natural disaster—unlike homeowner insurance companies, which must pay for losses caused by fires, floods, hurricanes and tornadoes, all increasingly common. The only global pandemic in our lifetime was caused by COVID-19. Given the dire public health ramifications, the US government responded by infusing billions of dollars into the healthcare system. Insurance companies paid more claims, but their losses were mitigated by those government subsidies. Their reserves were largely untouched, as was their revenue flow.

The considerable amount of money these companies squirrel away allows them to advertise on a large scale, even to the point of paying millions of dollars to have their name plastered on the ice of hockey stadiums or glued to the uniform of your favorite sports team. Personally, it makes my blood boil to see an insurance company logo on the left shoulder of the uniform of every player on my favorite baseball team. How all of that money, collected from premiums paid by patients and spent on advertising and executive perks, makes for better patient care is difficult to understand and is never explained in the insurance company's flashy and expensive media ads.

In the early days of medical insurance, medical care was not terribly expensive. Life expectancy was short, so patients didn't live long enough to develop chronic diseases. Prevention and screening were virtually nonexistent, so most people didn't enter the healthcare system until they were close to death. Technology was relatively primitive. If medicines didn't work, surgery was considered but there were no such things as minimally invasive procedures. Given the higher risks associated with open procedures, surgery was more of a last resort, and surgical volumes remained modest.

In relatively short order, medical science exploded in several specialties. It is impossible to list all the innovations that have been brought into common practice over the last twenty to thirty years, and that severely inflated costs. To mention a few, consider joint replacement surgery (now the most common operation in the elderly), fertility assessment and intervention, colonoscopy screening for colon cancer, cardiac catheterization, which began its life as a diagnostic tool but rapidly developed to intervention, CT and MR scanning and robotic and endoscopic surgery of several organs. While improving the quality of medical care, these new methodologies dramatically raised costs both by increasing the number of patients accessing them, and because the technology itself is expensive.

Genetic testing is a prime example of the current reimbursement insanity. Defining a genotype in a patient with one of a variety of diseases is imperative for several reasons. Besides empowering family counseling, it permits targeted therapy that increases the chances for therapeutic success. It also informs risk assessments by identifying individuals who may be more susceptible to drug side effects. Despite these acknowledged advantages, insurance companies are resistant to paying for genetic testing. They argue that in most cases, the information is not essential to patient management and doesn't contribute to better outcomes. The demand for genetic testing, like other technologies, has grown dramatically making insurance company roadblocks even more infuriating for clinicians who need the information to optimize patient care.

Compounding the growth and aging of the patient population is an exponential increase in the number of specialists trained to carry out high technology tests and procedures. Unfortunately, motivated by a flawed fee-for-service payment system, unprincipled physicians found ways to increase their volume of cases by testing or operating on patients who could easily have been managed more simply. In our patient example, remember that one of the options offered to Mrs. Dowd by Dr. Thom included cardiac catheterization. That test would have revealed a significant lesion in her coronary artery and Mrs. Dowd would have had a stent placed as a matter of course. However, in randomized clinical trials, patients with Mrs. Dowd's profile do just as well, with freedom from death or myocardial infarction, when managed aggressively with medications. These data have in no way stemmed the tide of expensive high-tech interventions. Coronary interventions increased rapidly, despite hard data that questions their utility.

The abuse of cardiac procedures is but one example of how improperly incentivized or poorly trained physicians have milked the medical care system over many years. Doctors have been creative in coming up with reasons to intervene and useless methods to do so. Whole companies have been formed to take advantage of an already overwhelmed medical care system. A prominent example is the use of stem cells to treat a variety of conditions such as arthritis without a scintilla of evidence of benefit. These unproven treatments place patients at considerable risk, as we saw in a recent case in which stem cell patients fell deathly ill from a bacterial contamination.

Profligate diversion of funds to worthless procedures means less money for neglected and important treatments, such as pre-natal care and childhood vaccinations.

The overuse of testing and intervention is also a consequence of the fear of litigation illustrated earlier in this book. Punishment for errors of omission is much more severe than those of commission, especially where diagnostic testing is concerned. Better to over-test and over-treat to keep the malpractice attorneys at bay. Had Dr. Thom sent Mrs. Dowd directly to catheterization, she would have had no liability, even if there had been a complication or a bad outcome. Dr. Thom got in trouble by trying to be a thoughtful and conservative professional.

The predictable result of the rise of technocracy and its warm embrace by unprincipled practitioners has been a dramatic increase in the overall cost of care. Spending on medical care in the US has reached absurd proportions, especially considering the poor return on the dollar. The US continues to trail all developed western nations when it comes to important healthcare outcomes like infant mortality and life expectancy, despite spending more per capita on healthcare than any other country on the planet.

To preserve their inappropriately large piece of the healthcare pie, insurers have adopted the speedbump strategy. If ordering tests and procedures is immensely difficult, insurance companies believe that practitioners will eventually become frustrated and order fewer of them. Pre-certification is the ruse. Practitioners are instructed to take an extra step and obtain assurance from the insurer that the test they are ordering is justifiable and will be reimbursed.

Precertification itself is a reasonable concept. For example, when in 1984 our research group proved that ordinary pacemakers were being implanted in patients who didn't need them, precertification became necessary for Medicare payment. The tactic was successful in reducing the inappropriate utilization of an expensive and invasive procedure.

But that is not the way it works today. Insurance companies deliberately torment doctors and their staff by placing callers on terminal hold, ignoring emails, and generally wasting their time. As we saw with Dr. Thom, the strategy is effective. Practitioners eventually give up and order a cheaper and, in Mrs. Dowd's case, a less accurate test just to move the process along. In addition to time-wasting, these obfuscations jeopardize good patient care. Physicians realize that they must work around the insurer to protect themselves against litigation (from which the insurer is immune) and, more importantly, to treat a patient in need. In the last vignette, unsuccessful appeals, including a frustrating and failed "peer-to-peer" plea for a drug for a suffering patient, led to an ablation the patient didn't need and which caused substantial harm.

CONCLUSION AND PATIENT ADVICE

As we will see many times in this compendium of cases, knowing the rules of engagement will help patients succeed in getting the medical care they need and deserve. In the world of pre-certification, doctors are relatively powerless. Yes, they can scream into the phone and send angry emails to insurers who deny their requests but, in the end, they have no leverage. There is a limited number of health insurance companies, and most of them are so large that a doctor who withdraws from their panel of providers out of frustration with their practices will soon have an empty office and be out of business. Unfortunately, our professional organizations have not succeeded in petitioning either the payers or the legislators to redress grievances. Calls for unionization to increase provider leverage have increased with some interesting developments, but the magnitude and breadth of the problems doctors face makes these initiatives look like mere guerilla warfare.

On the other hand, a complaining patient, especially one who is informed and ready to report a negligent insurance company to a state commissioner or a local congresswoman, or to post an unfavorable review on the internet, is more likely to succeed in getting the treatment she or he needs. Obviously, pulling out the stops to leverage a prescription for a therapy that is not important, or for which there really are less expensive alternatives, is not worthwhile. But pressing the insurer in situations where therapy decisions have a life-or-death impact, or a huge quality of life impact, as with Mrs. Dowd, is certainly worth the trouble and time. It requires a partnership with a doctor who can help by educating you about the rationale for your plea, and by providing the facts that substantiate your claim.

Story 7: Direct-to-Consumer Advertising and Other Drug Company Nonsense

"One of the missions of the practicing physician is to convince the masses of patients NOT to take medicine." —Sir William Osler

NARRATIVE

Mrs. West was a 68-year-old African American woman living in a historically Black metropolitan neighborhood with her husband. She had three children, all married and living in other parts of the country. She was a retired school cafeteria worker and an active member of her local community organization. She hadn't seen a doctor for a few years, but when she felt a lump in her breast a year ago, she scheduled an appointment at a university medical clinic. The medical resident who saw her with his attending physician confirmed that there was a single mass in her left breast, and he thought there were a few prominent lymph nodes in her armpit. They made a referral to a general surgeon for a biopsy, which confirmed a diagnosis of breast cancer that involved two lymph nodes. Fortunately, a bevy of scans found no evidence of spread to other organs. A mastectomy was performed without complications.

After recovering from surgery, Mrs. West was referred to the oncology clinic, where the consultant, Dr. Shah, saw her and recommended radiation and chemotherapy, just in case there was any cancer left in her body. The treatments went well. Mrs. West was nauseated and sick but relieved when the treatment cycles were completed after six months, and she could resume normal activity.

At her one-year visit, Dr. Shah delivered the bad news that during routine follow-up imaging, cancer was detected in her lungs and liver. She was given the option of further treatment but was told that the chances of extending her life substantially were slim. She promised to think about it and discuss options with her family.

A few days after she received this terrible news, Mrs. West and her husband were having dinner while watching the national news. One of the many healthcare commercials that aired that evening concerned what the product spokesperson continuously referred to as MBC, an acronym for metastatic breast cancer, or cancer that has spread from its primary site in the breast to one or several other organs in the body. Exactly Mrs. West's issue.

The product spokesperson began by reminding the TV viewers that MBC is associated with a poor prognosis and that treatment options are limited because women (and rarely men) with this disease have already exhausted multiple rounds of chemotherapy and radiation treatment.

But, according to the spokesperson, a new drug had just been approved that "offers real hope of living a longer life for women afflicted with MBC." Mrs. West watched as several expensively dressed, healthy-looking women with big smiles danced to lively music, hugging children, spouses and dogs. The spokesperson cheerfully detailed how wonderful this new treatment was, claiming it would "extend the life of women with MBC," giving them more time to enjoy life. Talking very fast and in a low voice, the spokesperson listed adverse events that had "happened" in the drug's clinical trials. Some of them sounded scary, including uncontrolled infections, seizures, heart attacks and even sudden death caused by a heart arrhythmia. But nothing seemed to affect the women in the commercial, or dimming their enthusiasm, as they continued their joyful activities unabated.

The narrator urged viewers who had MBC to "talk to your doctor" to find out if they might be a candidate for the drug. And finally, the spokesperson stated that the drug company might be able to provide discounts to make the drug "affordable" for the patient. Since it is not mandated, the actual cost of the drug was not part of the commercial.

A few days later, Mrs. West had her next appointment at the oncology clinic with Dr. Shah. She had written down the name of the drug and the company that was marketing it. When Dr. Shah solicited questions about her current situation or treatment, Mrs. West asked if he had heard of this new drug and what he thought of it.

Dr. Shah said he knew all about the new treatment and had considered recommending it for Mrs. West but hadn't for several reasons. First, Mrs. West didn't have the exact genetic profile of the women in the clinical trial for whom the drug had been approved. New cancer therapies are highly targeted to specific genetic types to maximize their efficacy. Therefore, there was no guarantee it would be effective for Mrs. West. Also, she had a history of mild high blood pressure, and Dr. Shah was concerned that if the drug depressed cardiac function as it was known to do, she might go into heart failure. Furthermore, the drug was very expensive, more than $50,000 for the first round of treatment, and the oncologist's experience with insurers was that they looked for every possible reason not to pay for it. The approval process could take weeks, time that Mrs. West didn't have. Finally, while it was true that the drug did prolong life, the average increase was about four to six months during which time patients could suffer from multiple side effects.

Given Mrs. West's profile, and weighing the pros and cons, Dr. Shah had determined she was not a good candidate for the new drug. However, if she and her husband were eager to try the new drug, he would see if her insurance company would approve it.

Mrs. West talked about it with her family and decided to give the medication a try. The approval process, however, moved at glacial speed. The insurance company requested several details, including the rationale for what they referred to as "off-label use," that is, use in a patient with a genetic profile different from that of the women in the drug's clinical trial. The insurance company also wanted to know exactly what therapy Mrs. West had received and failed, and information on her cardiovascular disease status. Dr. Shah attempted several times to enlist the help of the company that manufactured the drug, with the hope that the drug company would be able to leverage the balking payer or at least provide a discount if the insurance company didn't grant coverage. That strategy was not successful. The only concession from the drug company was the possibility of a 10 percent discount on the cost of the drug with the use of coupons that they would supply to the patient, but only after the insurance company approved its use.

After six weeks of wrangling, the insurance company agreed to pay for an initial round of treatment. Payment for further treatment cycles would depend on Mrs. West's progress and tolerance of the new drug. Mrs. West and her family were thrilled. During the long wait, her overall health had deteriorated to the point that she could no longer leave her home and spent most of her time in bed. Now, they finally had some hope.

The first intravenous infusion of the new drug occurred in Dr. Shah's office the following week and lasted about ninety minutes. It left Mrs. West weak and nauseated but able to return home. She spent most of the night in the bathroom, vomiting repetitively.

Over the next few days, as the effects of the drug slowly dissipated, Mrs. West began to get her strength back and was able to keep most food down. The following week was the best she had had in a long time. She was even able to spend some time with her grandchildren. Her oncologist was cautiously optimistic. His nurse practitioner even told Mrs. West that her decision to ask for the drug was reasonable, after all.

Which is why everyone was so disappointed and upset when, ten days after the first drug infusion, Mrs. West said good night to her husband and went to sleep, never to awaken.

CASE EXPLANATION

Mrs. West had end-stage breast cancer. The malignancy had spread to other organs, and she and her oncologist knew it was only a matter of time until she died of her disease. The search continues for treatments to prolong life for patients with metastatic breast cancer, but so far most have not had a significant impact on survival.

Mrs. West had a competent oncologist who had weighed the risks and benefits of the new therapy touted in the TV commercial and had decided not to prescribe it. Why didn't Dr. Shah offer the new treatment? His reasons were reasonable and rational. Physicians are charged with sorting through various treatment options and choosing the one most appropriate for the patient. This is called "individualization of care" and is fundamental to the art and practice of medicine. It could be argued that he should have discussed any possible new treatment with Mrs. West before putting the idea aside. "Shared decision making" is an important element in patient management. Had that conversation taken place before Mrs. West saw the commercial, her enthusiasm might have been dimmed, and the outcome different.

Mrs. West and her husband were desperate and decided to try a drug that they knew could be dangerous to the point of shortening her life or making her existence so unpleasant that the extra time would be a torment. They were clearly influenced by the TV commercial in which the benefits were overstated and the risks minimized. Nonetheless, her oncologist acquiesced. Dr. Shah, a good and caring oncologist, acknowledged that, given the dire nature of her disease, Mrs. West's decision to explore all options was reasonable.

As it happened, the oncologist had been correct to demur. The new treatment was known to influence the heart's electrical system, making it more prone to ventricular fibrillation, a heart rhythm incapable of sustaining heart function and circulation. In Mrs. West's case, the risk of a fatal outcome was substantial. Patients with high blood pressure develop thickened heart walls that render the heart more susceptible to going out of rhythm. Given the circumstances of her death, Mrs. West almost certainly had a lethal cardiac rhythm disturbance, exactly as the oncologist had feared. Mrs. West had taken a chance to extend her life by a few months, just as the TV commercial encouraged, but for her, the outcome was quite different. Perhaps she was lucky not to not have suffered a slow and agonizing death, but her sudden demise was a blow to her husband and everyone who loved her. They were deprived of their chance to say goodbye.

COMMENTARY

Pharmaceutical and medical device companies are in the business of making money for their shareholders. That is their primary mission. Companies espouse the idea that their goal is to help patients live longer and better lives, and it is true that the physicians and other scientists who work in industry are well intentioned and rightly motivated. They work hard, conducting developmental research to discover more safe and effective therapies for patients. However, that is not the prime directive of the company's officers. They answer to their board and the stockholders. Profits and stock prices are their highest priority.

New drug development is a complicated and costly process. The average cost to bring a new chemical entity from the lab bench to the clinic averages one to three billion dollars. After painstaking non-clinical research in experimental models, the drug can be introduced into normal volunteers, followed by a gradual introduction into the target population. The regulatory bar is high, especially for drugs or devices that carry a substantial risk of harm. Once approved, agreement for payment by insurers is the next hurdle, predicated on its value over and above what might already be available for its indication. This is followed by a campaign to market the drug to doctors and other healthcare providers. Very few drugs are commercially successful to the point of being "blockbuster" therapies that earn the developer billions more than their initial investment. But the search for the Holy Grail continues.

The amount of time a drug manufacturer has to recoup its investment in a new drug is limited by its patent life. Much of that time is eaten away during the long process of development and regulatory approval so companies frequently have less than five to ten years of exclusivity remaining at the time a new drug is launched. Once a successful new drug goes off patent, it is copied by several generic manufacturers. The new competition may help reduce the cost of the drug but not always, and not as much as a true free market would predict. Backroom deals among the many manufacturers and with the original patent holder can serve to keep the price up to optimize profits. Pharmacy benefit managers, the middlemen selling to retail pharmacies, take a healthy cut for themselves, further inflating the price.

Our government has encouraged generic drug development to control price, which it does to some extent, but there are issues. For a generic drug to be approved, it must be "bioequivalent" or "biosimilar." That means the amount of generic drug delivered must be similar, but not necessarily identical, to the brand drug. For most indications, similarity is acceptable. A generic headache pill having eighty percent of the potency of the original product is not a big deal. But for life-threatening conditions for which exact therapeutics is required, such as heart attack or stroke treatments, generic drugs may not measure up. Without head-to-head clinical trials comparing generic to brand drugs, we will never know for sure if efficacy and safety are really the same.

Another issue is general availability. Once a drug goes off patent, the original manufacturer may completely cease production and move on to new patentable agents. Depending on the potential profitability of the drug, only one or a few generic houses may continue producing it. These companies may be small with limited resources so if their production capability is suddenly compromised, for example with a production line problem, commonly used drugs may become completely unavailable for long periods of time. As you have seen in the news, this situation is now occurring with alarming frequency, placing patients in grave jeopardy. When drugs are scarce, physicians are encouraged by hospital administrators to limit their use to the most ill patients, or to substitute less effective or safe alternatives. As in most situations, if patients have a bad outcome because of these common drug shortages, physicians, not drug makers or administrators, will be blamed.

Ordinarily, marketing of medicines and devices is directed at providers who may prescribe a drug or implant a device based on what he or she is told by the advertiser, or what they know from the literature. Sales representatives are dispatched to hospitals and doctor offices to "detail" new therapies and hopefully motivate practitioners to try them. In recent years, this marketing strategy has become less effective because many healthcare systems have limited representatives' access to physicians. They do so to dissuade inappropriate use of new therapies spurred by glossy advertisements that are delivered by particularly attractive salespeople. In a subsequent vignette, we will see how these sales tactics can sidetrack good patient care.

Ironically, while doctor visitations have been choked off, industry has been granted the opportunity to advertise their products to the public through all media formats, including television, radio and print. Direct-to-consumer (DTC) advertising includes ads for prescription drugs and devices regardless of indication or their target population. The permission to air ads for drugs is nearly unique to the United States. Except for New Zealand, no other country in the world allows DTC advertising on the premise that the public cannot understand the intricacies of medical treatment and cannot select among the myriad of options available for most diseases. These countries have correctly concluded that DTC advertising is necessarily misleading. Though it may increase prescription rates, given the high cost of TV ads, it may also be a waste of money.

The cost of advertising is one explanation for the incredible difference in the price of drugs in the US compared to other First World countries, where comparator studies are required to demonstrate superiority over existing therapies to justify "premium pricing." However, there is another factor: the "middleman." Pharmacy Benefits Managers are responsible for the distribution of drugs to retail pharmacies and hospitals in the US. In the process, they inflate prices to increase their share of the already bloated revenue. Consider the fact that patients who could be candidates for generic drugs at a much lower cost are frequently provided with a brand equivalent that not only takes more out of their pockets but also places an enormous burden on an already strained healthcare system. Though operating in the shadows for years, exploitation of US drug marketing and distribution by these managers has recently been exposed. Whether and how these organizations will be brought under control is far from clear.

Despite how illogical and expensive it is, DTC advertising has taken hold in the US. Almost any TV program, especially the news viewed by an increasingly aging public, is peppered with commercials advertising everything from homeopathic and relatively worthless placebos all the way to complex treatments for rare diseases. And no disease is rare enough or private enough to be spared. Thus, the advertising blitz takes on Peyronie's disease (penile fibrotic distortion), Dupuytren contracture (crooked finger), pseudobulbar palsy (inappropriate emotional outbursts), and any number of diseases that blotch the skin, cause diarrhea, or bring on unpleasant odors from the nether regions. Medications for skin diseases are particularly popular. Who doesn't want to look like the beautiful people who used to have disfiguring rashes but are now free to wear skimpy outfits to show off their blemish-free skin?

Perhaps most disconcerting is that drug manufacturers have discovered that populating their commercials with famous athletes and entertainers enhances the credibility of their claims and stokes interest regardless their worth. While Shaquille O'Neal touts the value of Icy Hot, a skin gel to reduce arthritic pain, Magic Johnson encourages viewers to get vaccinated against RSV, and Kareem Abdul-Jabbar hawks blood thinners to prevent stroke in patients with atrial fibrillation.

The FDA is charged with regulation of drug and device advertising. A set of explicit rules applies, and all commercials are reviewed to ensure accuracy and balance. Claims of efficacy must conform entirely to what is stated in the brochure with directions for use that accompanies every new drug or device approval. If a drug relieves diarrhea, an actor or a real patient in a commercial can portray that benefit but no other. Encouraging off-label use is expressly prohibited. The commercial needs fair balance so all potentially serious side effects must be stated (but not necessarily portrayed), which is the reason for the rapidly spoken litany of warnings delivered by an unseen person on TV ads, and written in small print at the bottom of the screen. Violations of these regulations such as exaggeration of the magnitude of the treatment effect or understatement of the hazards, result in the immediate withdrawal of the commercial, not the product, and not necessarily a broadcast retraction.

What has emerged is a cascade of slickly produced ads intended to inspire enough patient interest and enthusiasm for a new drug to bring it up when they see their physicians. To some extent, the ads are educational, despite themselves. How many people knew their LDL cholesterol level or hemoglobin A1C concentration before they saw commercials promoting lipid lowering or anti-diabetes medications? Even healthcare providers say they learn things from commercials about new products that may be helpful in their practices. But, as with TV advertising in general, the actors and scenes are carefully orchestrated to emphasize the euphoria that comes with clear skin, less weight, lower blood pressure, or better diabetes control. In short, the idea is to raise expectations so that the guy sitting in his easy chair at home eating potato chips and drinking beer will ask for a drug that will make him look like and feel like the people in the commercial who just stepped out of *GQ*.

As for the downside risk, advertisers are required to list major side effects. To comply, they use medical terminology that even a medically trained audience would struggle to follow, at a pace that defies retention. Most people would have a hard time saying "multiple endocrine neoplasia syndrome type 2," let alone knowing enough to remind their doctors to rule it out before prescribing the latest diabetes treatment miracle. Or how about exocrine pancreatic insufficiency, a rare disease that allows companies to advertise and sell food-based treatments with unproven efficacy to anyone who has loose stools or gas because they simply have irritable bowels?

If you really pay attention, there should be a lot of things about these commercials that make you wonder. For example, how are you supposed to know if you are allergic to the medication unless you've already taken it? And if you did have an allergic reaction, what class of idiot would you need to be to ask your doctor to prescribe it again? And wouldn't you like to know a little more about the deaths that occurred in the clinical trial? Were they disease-related or were people hit by a bus? Isn't angioedema the side effect that can cause your throat to close, so you suffocate to death? What are the chances that will happen to you and if it did occur, what could you do about it?

The retort from the drug makers, of course, is that you have to talk to your doctor before you get the medication so all these issues can be explained in greater detail. But are they? How many doctors review all the possible side effects of a drug before prescribing it? And which of your many doctors are you supposed to talk to and ask these questions? And how often does the hapless primary care physician, seeing a patient every ten minutes, and without in-depth knowledge about the disease in question, cave in and prescribe whatever the patient asks for? And how often, as in Mrs. West's tragic case, does the knowledgeable doctor take pity and administer a futile therapy to preserve whatever hope a terminal patient has remaining? As we learned with laetrile, a worthless cancer treatment that patients traveled to Mexican clinics to obtain, desperate people will grasp at just about any straw no matter how ridiculous and unfounded.

If DTC prescription drug advertising to potential patients is an inane idea, think about the advertising of complicated medical devices. One company put on a multi-million-dollar campaign to tell patients they might want to talk to their doctor about getting an implanted defibrillator to prevent sudden death. "Ten thousand more hugs" from their grandchildren were in the offing if they had the procedure. Otherwise, they would likely not be around to receive them.

The enormity of a decision to implant a defibrillator in any patient is difficult to exaggerate. It is a life-changing event and is appropriate for only a small percentage of patients with heart disease. Implants carry substantial risk with the prospects of life-long device management. Furthermore, in this commercial, the company did not see fit to disclose that twelve to fourteen high-risk patients would need to have an implant to save one life, odds that many patients wouldn't want to take on. If the intent is to provide life-saving information to a wide patient audience, why don't manufacturers buy commercial time to inform patients when a device they carry around in their body and on which their life depends has been recalled by the FDA for a safety issue, as they frequently are? Doctors complained so bitterly about being deluged by inappropriate requests for a defibrillator, and the time they had to spend to disabuse patients of the need for it, that the manufacturer finally removed the commercials from the air.

But that didn't stop others who have advertised specialty devices for niche indications. Have you seen the commercial for a device to prevent blood clots from leaving the heart and going to the brain to cause a stroke in patients who have atrial fibrillation? After watching that commercial, do you have any idea of the benefit and risk, if you are a candidate, or how to go about making an informed decision? And why would you want to have that device implanted when Kareem Abdul-Jabbar already told you that he takes a pill that does a particularly good job of doing the same thing as the device in preventing a stroke? Is Kareem wrong, and if so, is the doctor who gave you the drug instead of the device somehow incompetent?

One of my colleagues spoke to me after seeing a patient who came in with questions about getting a heart valve that had been advertised on television to replace her leaking one. "Does this patient think I'm a moron?" she asked. "I guess if she thinks I need help from a TV commercial, it might be a good idea for her to find a smarter doctor."

As if DTC advertising of prescription drugs wasn't bad enough, the ads for non-prescription drugs are even more maddening. In this realm, there is almost no regulatory control. If a product is deemed a "food substance" or safe for non-prescription use, proof of efficacy can be as thin as having an individual patient proclaim that "this product worked for me." Since such products are largely impotent, side effects are not common, a fact emphasized in the commercials that promote them.

Given weak regulation and the possibility of exaggerated claims, there is great interest in designing and selling substances that are food derived and mostly safe, but unlikely to help. In these scenarios, it is all about marketing, coming up with catch words and phrases that resonate with potential users. Taking jellyfish extract can give you a "memory like an elephant," or if you have erectile dysfunction, we have a pill that "never fails to make your wife happy." One common phrase in these ads is "clinical studies have shown…" when the science referred to is likely a non-controlled trial in a small sample of non-relevant subjects carried out in a foreign country.

Why is the public so easily deceived into spending billions of dollars on worthless healthcare products? Clearly, there is a distrust of the medical care establishment, given the failures of many mainstream therapies that were touted to be safe and effective. It is much easier to go to the drug store and buy an over-the-counter erectile dysfunction drug than to confess to a healthcare provider that you can't achieve an erection. If your doctor has told you about a clinical trial proving that a specific formulation of fish oil reduces the chances of dying from heart disease, why pay hundreds of dollars for that drug if unproven doses and formulations can be purchased at the drug store for vastly less money? And going to a quack who injects stem cells or collagen into your joints seems more palatable than having joint replacement surgery with the pain and long rehabilitation associated with it, even if the injections lack solid proof of efficacy.

Most influential in prompting misguided patient decisions is the placebo effect. People who are convinced that the treatment they are taking is effective are likely to perceive benefit. Given the powerful effect of placebo, any study that purports to show improved quality of life cannot be evaluated without a placebo arm, an element that is almost always missing from the development of homeopathic drugs or devices. If someone you trust, like a retired football hero, says that doing something as ridiculous as wrapping a copper band around your waist will reduce back pain, you are likely to have less back pain when you buy one and put it on. How much of that improvement is an effect of the copper band, and how much is because of your faith in the football player, or your eagerness to find relief, or your refusal to believe you were bilked, is unknowable.

CONCLUSION

We owe a debt to pharmaceutical and device companies that have helped clinical scientists over many years develop new and effective treatments for a variety of important diseases. The partnership between academia and industry has been essential for much good science and improvement in patient care. However, once again, the opportunity to make a profit, especially a big profit, is corruptive. An increasing number of commercial firms without scientific and medical expertise have entered the medical care business. With the help of intense lobbying and in the name of an open capitalistic economy, drug and device companies have profited mightily. Prices for their products are outrageous, made even more so by the exorbitant costs of advertising them to inappropriate and naïve audiences. Consider that spending on drugs in the United States totaled $487 billion dollars in 2024, including $98 billion that came directly out of the patients' pockets. Citizens of all other First World countries paid exactly nothing.

I once thought that advertising complex therapies for serious diseases to an unschooled audience would ultimately prove to be futile and a big waste of money, and it would dry up. Drug companies may be greedy, but they aren't stupid. And yet, DTC advertising works. It is an effective way to sell more drugs and to make more money. What that tells us about the sophistication of patients and the wisdom of their physicians is not very palatable. In any case, DTC advertising will not go away unless outlawed, and commercials will be hard to ignore, especially if you have a serious disease that those happy actors on TV are battling successfully. Just remember that those highly touted panaceas will never work as well as you are being told, or as safely.

PATIENT ADVICE

As H. L. Mencken famously said, "For every complex problem, there is a solution that is simple, clear, and wrong." The message to patients is: Beware of cures that are advertised on TV as easy fixes to complex diseases. If plaque psoriasis or rheumatoid arthritis or amyloidosis or atrial fibrillation were as simply treated as implied in television commercials, our clinics would be empty. Your most important priority must be to identify and align with a physician you trust. Conversations about treatment alternatives should be part of the agenda of your visits with that person. Through an excellent therapeutic relationship with someone who can address your questions, you won't need to stay up to watch the eleven o'clock news to have Lady Gaga guide you in the best way to rid yourself of those damnable migraine headaches. And you won't have to wonder if a political sycophant with a worm in his brain knows what he is talking about when he tells you that vitamin A is better than a vaccine for preventing measles.

Story 8: Technology for its Own Sake

"In the sickroom, ten cents' worth of human understanding equals ten dollars' worth of medical science." —Martin Fischer

NARRATIVE

This story begins not with a patient but with a young and recently minted cardiologist, Dr. Gold, who had an interest in electrophysiology. She was trained to be an arrhythmia specialist at a prestigious East Coast institution by inspirational mentors. They offered her an opportunity to stay on as a junior attending physician at their university. After carefully considering their offer, Dr. Gold and her husband decided they were tired of big cities. Also, Dr. Gold didn't want to get on the treadmill and try to climb the rigid and misogynistic academic pyramid in which women were terribly undervalued and underpaid. She was attracted to the idea of living in a smaller city, where she could establish her own arrhythmia program and build it her way.

She entertained several offers and finally settled on a 150-bed community hospital in a medium-sized Midwest industrial town about eighty miles from that state's university medical center. The hospital president was excited about her recruitment and had made a generous offer of facilities and salary that would be contingent on performing a substantial number of cases. These incentives were not expected to be an issue because Dr. Gold's new electrophysiology program meant that the dozens of patients being referred every year to the university hospital for ablation procedures would now be retained, as would their hospital and professional fees.

As Dr. Gold learned, the process of setting up a new program and laboratory was complicated. It involved hiring and training nurses and other professionals to operate the laboratory, establishing an outpatient device clinic, and buying a myriad of equipment for the electrophysiology laboratory itself.

Dr. Gold was energized and worked hard during her first few months to get everything and everyone up to speed. As part of her preparation, she decided to attend the national scientific meetings of the arrhythmia society of which she was a brand-new member. At that meeting, every company selling electrophysiology laboratory equipment had a technical exhibit in an area the size of a small city. Each booth was populated by expert salespeople who would help Dr. Gold sort through her many options and begin to decide which machines would be best for her new electrophysiology laboratory. There was also a job bureau where skilled ancillary professionals could be found and recruitment begun.

Because electrophysiological procedures involve the insertion of catheters into the heart, one of the important items for purchase was X-ray equipment. Fluoroscopy is used to follow the movement of catheters through the body from their insertion site in peripheral veins and arteries to specific areas of the heart. The equipment is expensive but sophisticated, providing high quality images while limiting the amount of radiation to which the patient and staff might be exposed. The company marketing the equipment that Dr. Gold finally selected included installation and staff training as part of their purchase price.

To Dr. Gold's relief, all went well with the acquisition, shipment and installation of the equipment she had ordered. Besides fluoroscopy, various devices for the stimulation, recording, and processing of the heart's electrical signals were installed, while the staff received intensive instruction on the use of each component. After everything was in place, the state's department of health conducted an inspection and deemed the laboratory safe and ready for its first clinical case.

Dr. Gold thought that it would a good idea to make the first case a relatively easy one that wouldn't tax the staff or the facilities. She chose a 48-year-old man with a relatively simple form of tachycardia called AV nodal reentry. That means the patient had been born with an extra electrical pathway within the junction box or node that carried signals from the top chambers to the bottom chambers of the heart. When a premature beat from the top chamber arrived at the node, it could touch off a tachycardia, a rapid heart action that would make the patient weak and breathless until it stopped on its own or was terminated, usually by an intravenous drug in the emergency department.

AV nodal reentry is a relatively common condition that can be treated with medication. However, the problem can be cured by ablating or cauterizing the extra pathway in the AV node, the so-called slow pathway. The procedure is relatively straightforward and safe. Ablation would consist of applying radiofrequency energy to cauterize and destroy the extra pathway. Dr. Gold would make detailed recordings during the procedure to locate the pathway and then eliminate it. Like most with this condition, her inaugural patient had an otherwise normal heart and would easily handle the stress of the procedure.

The patient, Mr. Lee, had had two episodes of tachycardia that required emergency room visits and several shorter ones that stopped on their own. Since he traveled quite a bit and spent time in airplanes, he was eager to be rid of the problem and not have to worry about a recurrence when he wasn't close to medical care. He readily agreed to having an ablation procedure, even though he understood that the arrhythmia was not life-threatening. He decided that an ablation was a reasonable option, better than taking medication on a continuing basis to suppress the extra electrical pathway.

Dr. Gold explained to Mr. Lee that she could do the ablation right there in his home hospital without the need to be referred to another institution. She was confident that the procedure would be successful and could be carried out safely. If all went well, the ablation would be a same-day procedure. Mr. Lee would arrive in the morning and go home in the afternoon when his anesthesia wore off. Mr. Lee was pleased with the arrangements, agreed to go forward, and the laboratory's first case was scheduled.

At 6 a.m. on the day of the procedure, Mr. Lee arrived at the hospital's pre-surgical unit and went through the customary preparations, including meeting an anesthesiologist. He wasn't going to be put under general anesthesia, rather a lighter anesthetic would be used to make sure he was mostly asleep and comfortable during the procedure while being monitored carefully by the anesthesiologist and her staff. Dr. Gold came by to greet him as well, to answer any final questions, and to reassure him of an excellent outcome.

Mr. Lee was then brought into the electrophysiology laboratory and given a sedative to help him relax while he was transferred to the procedure table and drapes applied. Just as Dr. Gold came into the lab, the head nurse approached to tell her that the technician responsible for operating the fluoroscopy equipment had called in sick. Dr. Gold asked if there was anyone else who could run the X-ray equipment. Dr. Gold was particularly concerned because she herself had not been trained extensively in that area, and she would have to rely on the staff's expertise. The head nurse reassured her that all the lab technicians had attended the X-ray equipment training sessions and that they should be good to proceed with a substitute at the controls of the X-ray equipment.

No matter how much preparation and training, inaugural cases are always more difficult than anticipated. Though Dr. Gold had performed dozens of AV node modifications as a fellow in training, she struggled mightily with her first unsupervised procedure. Mr. Lee did have an extra pathway in his AV node as she had suspected, but the abnormal slow pathway sat very close to the normal fast one. Dr. Gold was concerned that if she applied heat energy too close to the normal pathway, Mr. Lee would develop heart block and require a pacemaker, not a good outcome by any means.

Dr. Gold worked for two hours, using fluoroscopy to reposition the catheter and delivering low energy test lesions. Given the length of the procedure, she asked the anesthesia staff to use propofol so that Mr. Lee would be fully asleep and not uncomfortable on the table. He snored peacefully for the duration of the procedure.

Dr. Gold was finally able to obliterate the culprit pathway. She almost cried out in relief when it was clear that the procedure was successful. The tachycardia could no longer be initiated with artificially delivered premature stimuli. Mr. Lee awakened to get the good news before he was taken to the recovery suite. As Dr. Gold left the laboratory, she complimented the staff, remarking that the clarity of the X-ray images during the case was excellent, so much better than what she had been accustomed to in her training.

After speaking with Mrs. Lee and writing post-procedure orders, Dr. Gold was having a celebratory lunch with her team in the hospital cafeteria when she was summoned to the recovery area. Mr. Lee had a normal rhythm and blood pressure but was complaining of severe back pain.

Dr. Gold's first concern was a hemorrhage in the area behind the abdominal cavity called the retroperitoneum. Had the passage of the catheters perforated a large vessel? But when the nurse rolled Mr. Lee over, Dr. Gold discovered a large area of redness on his back with just the beginning of blistering in its center. Her first thought was that he was having an allergic reaction to the sheets or the gown he was wearing. She ordered Benadryl, an antihistamine, and steroid cream. The discomfort eased up and so after he was fully recovered, Mr. Lee was discharged with instructions to return to Dr. Gold's office for an evaluation in a week.

But only three days after discharge, Dr. Gold received a call from the emergency room. Mr. Lee was there because the steroid cream was no longer working, the rash on his back was significantly worse, and severe pain was keeping him awake at night. Dr. Gold asked the ER physician if there was a dermatologist on call who could see Mr. Lee in consultation. Since emergency dermatology consultation is not a common event, it took the ER physician a couple of hours to find someone who was willing to leave his office practice to see the patient in the ER.

Dr. Gold arrived in the ER just as the dermatologist was coming out of the exam bay with a worried look on his face. Dr. Gold introduced herself and asked for his opinion.

"Well, I can't say I have a lot of experience with radiation burns, but that sure looks like one to me."

Dr. Gold was aghast. "Are you sure?"

"No, I'm not sure, but I understand this guy was in your lab a few days ago and had fluoroscopy. The location of the burn and its shape suggests he had a radiation overdose from your image intensifier."

Dr. Gold began an investigation of the electrophysiology lab procedure. To her horror, she discovered that the technician who was operating the X-ray equipment for the procedure had misread the instructions and had inadvertently dialed up needlessly high radiation doses. That Mr. Lee had received a massive X-ray dose was confirmed by the fact that the radiation badges of those who had been in the room during the procedure, including Dr. Gold, had readings much higher than expected, grossly exceeding what would be considered a usual exposure. It also explained why the X-ray images were so clear and easy to interpret during the case.

Dr. Gold spoke with Mr. Lee, who was very upset to hear about a potential radiation overdose but agreed to be admitted to the hospital to receive intensive skin treatment. Dr. Gold apologized and assured him he would receive the best of care, including consultations to estimate his risk of malignancy and measures that could be taken to reduce the risk and keep him under surveillance. He was discharged a few days later with several treatments and prescriptions and provisions for home healthcare, gladly paid for in full by the worried hospital administrators. However, over the next few weeks, Mr. Lee's burn worsened to the point that he began to slough skin and develop painful ulcers at the edges of the wound. Despite multiple operations and skin grafts over the next several months, he was left severely scarred. In addition, no matter how many consultants were called in to help, he would carry a high risk of cancer for the rest of his life, just like the Hiroshima/Nagasaki survivors.

The hospital's risk management department advised Dr. Gold to maintain contact with Mr. Lee and to emphasize that they would pay for all his medical care and expenses as he recuperated. However, as time went by, her calls to Mr. Lee were not answered nor did he continue his appointments with her in the clinic. As they expected, the hospital and Dr. Gold were sued, and since there was no defense, the case was quickly and discreetly settled for a few million dollars, money that would in no way diminish Mr. Lee's agony, or that of Dr. Gold. The laboratory continued to operate for a few months, but referrals for ablation became increasingly infrequent as word of the catastrophe leaked out. The hospital president eventually decided to buy out Dr. Gold's contract and close the electrophysiology laboratory permanently. Dr. Gold and her husband relocated to parts unknown.

CASE EXPLANATION

Several important issues are illustrated by this case. Dr. Gold was a well-trained but novice electrophysiologist who possessed the skill to do ablation procedures but had no organizational experience. Left to her own devices, and incentivized to carry out revenue-generating procedures, she hastily built a laboratory that was not safe. A more experienced program leader would have put into place several fail-safe mechanisms to prevent patient harm, including the availability of trained replacement staff. She also showed poor judgment by proceeding with an elective procedure that could have easily been rescheduled for a time when all of her laboratory staff was available.

Mr. Lee had an arrhythmia that can be treated successfully with ablation. He wanted to be "cured" mainly because of his fear of having the arrhythmia when he didn't have access to prompt medical treatment. Anxious to launch her new electrophysiology lab, Dr. Gold encouraged Mr. Lee to have the procedure. However, Mr. Lee's attorneys in the lawsuit emphasized that Dr. Gold had not apprised Mr. Lee of the availability and effectiveness of medical treatment. Beta-blockers and calcium channel blockers can be used for arrhythmias like Mr. Lee's. Those drugs can be not only used constantly, but in some cases, intermittently to terminate the arrhythmia on demand to avoid an emergency room visit. Dr. Gold had not taken the time to document that balanced discussions with Mr. Lee had occurred. His attorneys made it look as if he had been railroaded into having a dangerous procedure without being offered reasonable alternatives.

Mr. Lee's attorneys also emphasized in their complaint that Dr. Gold had not informed the patient of the inexperience of the staff who performed his procedure. They claimed he had no idea his was the inaugural case at that hospital and that no one in the lab that day had ever assisted with an ablation procedure. Furthermore, he wasn't told that the technician who knew the most about the X-ray equipment was absent because of illness, and that lesser trained individuals would be at the controls.

Catheter ablation of the slow pathway in the AV node, as in Mr. Lee's case, may be "simple" in the minds of experienced operators, but like all invasive procedures, it carries risk. Dr. Lown, who was always wary of the overutilization of technology, used to tell me that when a physician refers a patient for an operation or catheterization, it is very much like sending that person into a minefield. Though the odds of stepping on a landmine may be small, if your patient is unlucky, the consequences can be dire and their injuries your fault.

The most frequent complication of AV node ablation is inadvertent ablation of both pathways, producing complete heart block, or inability to conduct impulses from the heart's normal pacemaker in the atria down to the main pumping chambers, the ventricles. What results is a very slow and unreliable heart rhythm that can be treated only by inserting a permanent cardiac pacemaker with its attendant maintenance and complications. Ironically, it was the fear of this complication that had caused Dr. Gold to spend extra time in the laboratory moving catheters under X-ray guidance. That translated into an increased fluoroscopy time that, along with high radiation doses, ultimately caused harm.

Any time that catheters are inserted into the heart, there is the potential for trauma to the vessels or the heart itself. Poking a hole in the heart or a major vessel can be catastrophic and is the reason why Dr. Gold first thought that Mr. Lee's back pain may have been caused by blood leaking from a damaged vessel into the retroperitoneal space. It can also result in pericardial tamponade, in which blood from a heart rupture leaks into the space between the heart muscle and its lining, squeezing the heart and not allowing it to fill and contract normally. This is a life-threatening complication that requires immediate treatment by sticking a needle through the chest wall into the pericardial space and draining the collected blood.

X-ray imaging is potentially dangerous if not administered correctly. Mr. Lee's case represents an extreme example of an overdose, but the number of people who staff catheterization laboratories and have unnecessary radiation exposure and subsequent harm is unknown. There clearly is an increased incidence of several forms of cancer in cardiac laboratory workers, despite the measures taken for radiation protection such as lead-lined barriers placed around the patient. High volume laboratories now limit radiation dose by using alternative forms of imaging like ultrasound for catheter manipulation, but these practices have not gained widespread acceptance. In addition, radiation in the laboratory mandates lead aprons for lab personnel. The extra weight places immense stress on the back and lower extremities, which explains the high incidence of back and joint maladies in people who work in cardiac laboratories, and the fact that many electrophysiologists retire early because of intractable back and hip pain.

Mr. Lee's injuries were particularly egregious. Besides the harm to his back that would take years to mitigate, the long-term higher risk of cancer in such a young person is difficult to countenance. Any monetary compensation was inadequate justice in his case.

In the end, Dr. Gold's elaborate laboratory was a bust. It is difficult to know if it would have thrived but for the extreme first case complication that became widely publicized to potential referring physicians and patients alike. The money that had been spent on equipment and staff would have to be absorbed by the already economically stressed community hospital that was in desperate need of nurses and space for their core business. Therefore, how badly Dr. Gold's misadventure negatively affected the care of hospital patients in the years to follow would be difficult to calculate.

COMMENTARY

Technology is seductive. People who go into medicine are easily influenced by the great number and variety of machines that have become an integral part of patient care. As they progress in their training, they are highly motivated to learn how to do procedures, especially those using high technology. There are several rewards for doing so, some monetary, some ego-boosting, and some because manipulating catheters and ablating arrhythmias can be just plain fun. To carry out a successful high-tech procedure is entirely gratifying and once a trainee gets the scent, it may be difficult to moderate.

In addition, technology impresses patients. Many believe that a center that has cutting-edge equipment necessarily delivers a higher quality of care. That's why TV commercials for hospitals emphasize patient accessibility to "state-of-the-art technology," taking the viewer on a virtual tour of facilities packed with glitzy equipment. What is necessarily missing from these advertisements is any idea of how experienced their operators are and how good their outcomes.

This story uses catheter ablation as an illustration, but examples of excessive use of technology abound. As one of my cynical attending physicians once remarked, "When you go to Midas, you get a muffler." He meant that referral to a procedural specialist has a high likelihood of culminating in an operation of some kind. Consider the science of sleep. During my entire career, I never had a snoring patient who was referred to a sleep center and not labelled as having sleep apnea and at serious risk of death. It is important to understand that snoring is ubiquitous but actual cessation of breathing caused by airway obstruction is not. Getting diagnosed with sleep apnea is not a trivial matter since the only proven effective treatment is a bulky, inconvenient CPAP mask, prescribed to be worn indefinitely. Its benefit is to help patients sleep better and have less daytime drowsiness, but it has never been shown to prolong life in any population. Use of such a device for patients who do not have severe sleep apnea is inappropriate, uncomfortable and expensive, and yet another example of profligate use of technology to enhance revenue.

More alarmingly, even when hard scientific data prove that non-interventional approaches are as good as or better than a procedure, doctors continue to intervene as if nothing new was learned. Witness the rise of coronary intervention for patients with angina pectoris or coronary insufficiency. Treatment for this condition can be medicines to improve coronary blood flow or to reduce oxygen requirements of the myocardium, versus coronary artery bypass surgery or catheter interventions to open the artery and place stents. Several large, long-term, well-conducted, randomized clinical trials have proven that medical treatment is perfectly satisfactory for most patients who lack accelerating or unstable symptoms, yet the number of catheter procedures in the US for stable coronary artery disease continues to grow exponentially.

What drives this insanity? Once again, follow the money trail. Hospitals generate enormous revenue for procedures and little, if anything, for medical treatment. Thus, the number of hospitals with catheterization laboratories has increased dramatically over the past few decades as small hospitals attempt to stem the referral of patients to larger academic institutions. It used to be that the availability of open-heart surgery in the hospital was a prerequisite for the establishment and support of a catheter intervention program. This would allow prompt bypass grafting in those cases in which a coronary artery closed during catheter manipulation. Now, however, the cardiac surgery requirement has been lifted and nearly any sized hospital can, almost without exception, open a catheterization laboratory with the intention of attracting enough cases to pay for itself and more.

Similarly, doctors are paid well for procedures, much better than when they talk to or examine patients in the office. Those whose practices are owned by health systems, which is a sharply increased percentage of physicians nationally, are heavily incentivized to keep the hospital laboratory humming with cases, or else they will need to find another job. Almost fifty percent of hospitals in the US already operate in the red so for them, generating procedure revenue is essential. How can we expect a physician, working under pressure, to make a balanced and rational decision about the best treatment course for a patient?

And the bias to use technology is not restricted to invasive procedures. Imaging has become a cash cow for doctors and hospitals alike. Whereas simple stress testing can be carried out economically and with a good yield, cardiologists insist on using advanced imaging in routine stress testing without compelling evidence of its added value. How much better is positron emission tomography scanning or magnetic resonance imaging than common ultrasound imaging during stress testing to obtain valid results? The answer from clinical trials is that these high-priced imaging procedures are marginally better at best, but the slightest advantage is enough to encourage widespread use of expensive technology. Hospital administrators are persuaded to purchase expensive equipment to be able to say in television commercials that they offer "cutting edge" treatments, even when their additive value is clearly marginal. This is especially true for smaller hospitals struggling to maintain market share in highly competitive metropolitan markets.

Consider that the country that spends the most on this high technology, the United States, has no better, and in some cases, worse outcomes from common diseases for which invasive techniques are used. Mortality rates from heart disease are not one iota higher in Canada compared with the US, even though the Canadians perform a fraction of the procedures and operations per capita. This profligate use of advanced technology goes on while funding to support simple and important interventions in the community, like childhood vaccination, pre-natal care and blood pressure and diabetes treatment, go begging. We hemorrhage money on advanced medical care with marginal benefit, delivered to the economically privileged.

Most distressing is the failure to regulate. The FDA is not empowered to enter cost effectiveness into any of its decisions about drug or device approvals. The federal government has no mechanism to limit the cost of any medical product. The Centers for Medicare and Medicaid Services (CMS), which has Medicare cost and purchasing oversight, can only approve or disapprove payment for drugs and devices. The price point is whatever the industry sponsor decides, take it or leave it. And with a snake oil salesman who has touted the value of worthless remedies now placed in charge of all Medicare payments at CMS, the likelihood of effective regulation is nil.

As illustrated in this story, there is practically no effective oversight of new healthcare facilities. Hospitals do have to file for permission to establish a new lab or imaging facility, but denials are rare, and almost never because yet another catheterization lab, for example, is unnecessary in a highly populated area. The idea of establishing an ablation laboratory in a 150-bed hospital within driving distance from an established center, as in this story, was absurd, but no one with any regulatory authority stood in the way.

What has led us to this ridiculous situation of having off-the-charts healthcare spending without adequate return? Politicians are reluctant to anger any segment of their constituency, hospitals included, for fear of retribution at the polls. Strong lobbies also argue for the freedom of healthcare institutions to make their own decisions about facilities. Republican-controlled state legislatures still adhere to the Reagan ideology of deregulation. Monitoring of facilities and operators for safe and effective outcomes is an old idea that has been implemented in a piecemeal fashion in the United States. Newspaper publication of surgical mortality and morbidity statistics for hospitals and individual operators gained momentum in the last decade but reports now are sporadic and not well publicized. Instead, with passage of the Sunshine Act, we now spend hundreds of millions of dollars keeping track of how much money doctors receive from industry for research and education, an exercise that has not had any proven impact on the quality of medical care or physician practice. Most patients don't even know that such a data set exists and don't care if their doctors provide consultation, as long as they do a good job of making them well.

Just because a hospital can do a given procedure doesn't mean that is where you should have it done. We know that procedures are usually carried out more successfully and safely in facilities that have higher volumes but there are many exceptions to that principle. Not all baseball players carry a .350 batting average. Similarly, not all doctors can be expected to use technology with the same skill. Ask Mr. Lee.

CONCLUSION

When patients are asked what constitutes a good doctor, most answers reference the professional's ability to communicate effectively. Experience factors in, as does a reputation for technical excellence, but the latter is much harder to quantify. Despite this finding, modern medicine has deemphasized bedside skills, such as history taking, physical examination and personal interaction, and glorified high technology. It has done so with little to no evidence that the extravagant use of technology adds substantially to better outcomes, but only to the erosion of confidence in our profession. Consider the fact that doctors are no longer the most respected professionals, ranking below nurses, engineers, veterinarians, dentists, and pharmacists. Getting that lost admiration and respect back will be a difficult task if we don't stop our foolish rush to technology for its own sake.

PATIENT ADVICE

For the patient-consumer, finding a place to have an operation or an invasive procedure is complicated. Though some data exist in the public domain, much of it is biased. Consider, for example, how much better are the outcome statistics for a center that refuses to operate on very sick patients versus a tertiary referral site that routinely takes those patients on. We have learned that television commercials are intentionally misleading, with self-aggrandizement the order of the day. There is nothing to stop any hospital or practitioner from saying anything they wish about their services, expertise, reputation or outcomes.

Leaning on a learned intermediary is as important here as in many of our other stories. Many different people can serve in this role. A nurse or a medical office worker, one you trust, is likely to have knowledge about the best places to obtain competent medical care and can provide good advice.

However, finding the right doctor who can effectively integrate a caring and thoughtful approach to management with effective and skillful use of technology is the ultimate goal. Such individuals do exist, mainly in the senior doctor generation that is now passing the baton to its successors. The question to be answered is whether newer generations of physicians will emulate compassionate thinkers and careful professionals or be seduced into an algorithmic, technocratic, cookie-cutter world of medicine, and in so doing create a quagmire into which our children and grandchildren will ultimately sink.

Story 9: Regulatory Failings and the Billion-Dollar Alternative Medicine Mess

"Doctors put drugs of which they know little into bodies of which they know less for diseases of which they know nothing at all." —Attributed to Voltaire

NARRATIVE

Mr. McCabe was an overall good guy. A 73-year-old Caucasian man who worked as a stock trader for years before retiring a few years earlier, he had kept himself in good shape and had no major medical illnesses. Which is why he was taken aback when, during a routine appointment with his family doctor, he was told his heart was out of rhythm. He insisted he had no symptoms and had noticed no diminution in his exercise capacity.

An electrocardiogram in the office confirmed that he was in atrial fibrillation, a common chaotic upper chamber arrhythmia that causes the heart to function less efficiently. His heart rate, blood pressure and the rest of his physical examination were normal. His primary care doctor recommended consultation with a cardiologist. Mr. McCabe agreed and three days later he saw an arrhythmia specialist who ordered a battery of tests to exclude a metabolic cause, and to rule out the presence of significant heart disease. Mr. McCabe was told that his heart was functioning well and that his thyroid tests and other metabolic parameters were normal.

The cardiologist told Mr. McCabe that he would live longer if he were placed back into normal rhythm. He was started on Coumadin (brand name for warfarin), the only oral blood thinner available at that time, to prevent a clot from leaving the heart and causing a stroke. He was also placed on a beta blocker to keep his heart rate under control.

There followed a series of medications and procedures that were unsuccessful in restoring and maintaining normal rhythm, including a catheter ablation procedure. The cardiologist was frustrated but undaunted and recommended a referral to a surgeon who might be able to help by combining a second catheter ablation on the inner surface of the heart with lesions placed on the outer surface through surgical incisions. It was called a "hybrid procedure" that helped some people with recalcitrant arrhythmias to stay in normal rhythm. When Mr. McCabe asked about the risks of the procedure, he was told that some of them were serious, but there was little choice. If he didn't try the hybrid procedure, his arrhythmia would become "permanent," and he would have to take blood thinners and other medications for the rest of his shortened life.

Mr. McCabe finally agreed to have the procedure, but he was despondent. His retirement was being ruined by this lingering and serious heart problem. He became depressed and stopped exercising and playing golf. His wife described him as impossible to live with. For months, their lives were miserable.

One day at breakfast, Mr. McCabe's wife reminded him of a friend he had played golf with years before they moved south. Wasn't he a rhythm specialist? she asked. Maybe Mr. McCabe should reach out to him for another opinion before going under the knife.

Mr. McCabe called his old friend, Dr. Nuff and was immediately invited to come north for a consultation. He was reminded to bring all his records with him for a thorough review. Their reunion was a happy one, each remembering the many rounds of bad golf they had played together at some nice courses. Dr. Nuff then listened carefully as Mr. McCabe related his story. Dr. Nuff asked his old friend several times if he had experienced any symptoms such as shortness of breath or lightheadedness. Mr. McCabe insisted that he felt well generally but was having a hard time mentally dealing with this new health challenge. After performing a thorough examination, Dr. Nuff left the examination room for several minutes to go through Mr. McCabe's records while the patient/friend waited nervously.

Dr. Nuff returned to the consultation room with a smile on his face. "I think I have a way forward for you," he said and began a detailed summary of what he had gleaned from the records.

In essence, he agreed that Mr. McCabe had a case of what was known as "lone atrial fibrillation" or AF without any other structural heart disease. He also agreed that the arrhythmia was having no serious adverse effect on Mr. McCabe's function and, for that reason, remaining in the arrhythmia over the long term would be a realistic option, as long as Mr. McCabe took a blood thinner and rate-control medications, as currently prescribed. In short, nothing more needed to be done.

Mr. McCabe was incredulous. If what Dr. Nuff said was true, why had his doctors in Florida put him through so many drug tests and procedures and even proposed surgery? Dr. Nuff reassured Mr. McCabe that there was hard scientific evidence from several randomized clinical trials that he could do very well while remaining in AF. Furthermore, there were no data to prove his life would be shortened as long as he had careful clinical supervision. He told Mr. McCabe this was another example of a risky procedure avoided with good clinical judgment and plain old common sense.

Dr. Nuff agreed to write a letter to his friend's doctors in Florida with his opinion. Mr. McCabe's management from that point on should be simple and uncomplicated. Mr. McCabe thanked Dr. Nuff for his expertise and returned to Florida, overjoyed that his active life and sense of well-being had been restored.

Three years went by, and Mr. McCabe remained well and fit. His doctors reluctantly agreed to provide follow-up care, although they reminded him at every visit that ablation was advancing, and he might want to reconsider his decision to remain out of rhythm. Mr. McCabe refused, happy to take his medications on schedule. He was ecstatic that the drugs used to moderate his heart rate and his anticoagulant had caused no problem whatsoever. His blood pressure and heart rate were controlled, and echocardiograms showed that his heart function remained normal. His INRs, the measurement of how thin his blood was with warfarin, remained rock stable. Life was good.

Mr. McCabe's wife was, like him, very active. She attributed her good health to regular exercise and to various supplements she took daily. She suggested to her husband that he take some of them to improve his stamina. Mr. McCabe could only chuckle, reassuring her that he felt well, while admitting that his ability to walk the golf course had waned as birthdays passed. On impulse, at his next cardiology visit, he asked the nurse practitioner who saw him if using supplements would be acceptable. She reassured him that they were unlikely to be harmful and might have some benefit. No harm in trying, she said confidently.

Mr. McCabe's wife recommended he start with olive leaf extract. She believed it had been particularly helpful. Mr. McCabe did an online search and could find nothing that sounded alarming. Several people, including his wife, had posted on Facebook that it had improved their energy levels, and even their sexual function, with absolutely no side effects.

Mr. McCabe started with two capsules daily and, to his surprise, he did feel more energetic, and he tolerated the extract well. All was splendid until one night when he rose from bed and went into the dark bathroom to urinate. His stream seemed sluggish and when he flicked on the light, he saw not urine in the toilet, but blood. He awakened his wife and asked her to take him to the emergency room.

In the ER, Mr. McCabe reported no urinary symptoms such as burning or frequency, which might have indicated a common infection. The results of Mr. McCabe's physical examination were normal, as were his lab tests—except for his INR value. It had been 2 to 3 for the past several readings, but now it was 13. This extremely high value meant that his blood was grossly overly thinned. He was treated with vitamin K and fresh frozen plasma to reverse the effects of warfarin and admitted for observation. He continued to bleed heavily for several hours and required four blood transfusions to maintain his blood pressure and to keep his heart rate from going too high. With the lowering of his INR, the bleeding continued for three days and then gradually stopped.

The hospital physicians were in a quandary, unable to understand the cause of the suddenly elevated INR. A battery of imaging studies revealed no urinary tract pathology, which meant that the high INR itself was the cause of the bleeding. But why had the INR suddenly skyrocketed?

When a senior medical student stopped by to talk to Mr. McCabe, he asked several detailed questions that no one else on the medical team had brought up. One was a request for a complete list of all of Mr. McCabe's medications, including supplements. Mr. McCabe related that he had recently started taking olive leaf extract with the permission of his physician's nurse practitioner. The student pulled out his phone and his impromptu medical literature search yielded a handful of case reports documenting patients on warfarin who bled heavily while taking olive leaf extract. The authors of the reports hypothesized an adverse drug interaction by which olive leaf inhibited the metabolism of warfarin, dangerously raising its levels and thus the intensity of anticoagulation. None of these case reports had been published in mainstream medical journals or in the popular press, and the association was therefore poorly appreciated.

Mr. McCabe survived the crisis. After his urinary bleeding had completely resolved, he was changed over to a new anticoagulant known to carry a lower risk of bleeding, while less susceptible to adverse drug interactions. He forgave his wife and the nurse practitioner but swore to both that his days of taking supplements were over.

CASE EXPLANATION

Mr. McCabe fell victim to a troubling problem, a life-threatening medical condition caused by a "harmless" supplement. How often this occurs is impossible to estimate, but those of us who prescribe drugs live in constant fear that one of our patients will use a substance that has an uncertain but significant interaction with one of the legitimate medications we have prescribed.

Warfarin, and anticoagulants in general, are particularly problematic because they have what is known as a "narrow therapeutic window." That is, it only takes a small change in their concentration in the body to cause either inadequate blood thinning that can lead to a stroke, or excessive thinning that can cause catastrophic bleeding. The nurse practitioner who answered Mr. McCabe's question about the safety of olive leaf extract failed to consider that he was taking an anticoagulant. Furthermore, she had no way of knowing that warfarin metabolism could be altered by olive leaf extract and therefore had no reason to prohibit its use.

Warfarin and other anticoagulants have complicated pharmacology, including their metabolism in the liver. Under ordinary circumstances, if physicians prescribe one of many drugs that can raise the INR by inhibiting liver enzymes, more frequent INR sampling is carried out to make sure the blood is not overly thin, which causes abnormal bleeding. Home INR testing is now common, so patients can check their INR values every day if necessary and inform their healthcare provider who can alter or discontinue offending interacting drugs. In Mr. McCabe's case, what happened to the INR was not predictable. The medical literature contained no systematic information about drug-drug interactions between warfarin and olive leaf extract. Mr. McCabe's increase in INR was not detected until it had risen to levels never seen in that hospital's laboratory.

Mr. McCabe was fortunate. He was able to get to an emergency facility quickly, his problem was rapidly recognized and diagnosed, and reversal agents, antidotes and blood products were administered promptly so he didn't bleed to death or suffer other complications of massive blood loss such as a stroke or heart attack. If he had been older or had had disease in his coronary or cerebral vessels, as most people who use anticoagulants do, a catastrophic event such as bleeding into his brain, would have been more likely.

Mr. McCabe's case occurred just as new oral anticoagulants were being introduced. He was eventually transitioned to one of them to keep him safe, but would they? It is true that in head-to-head, blinded, randomized trials, the new DOACs (direct acting oral anticoagulants) have been associated with less bleeding than warfarin and, in some cases, better effectiveness in preventing strokes and death in patients with atrial fibrillation. Unfortunately, like warfarin, they are also subject to drug interactions that can increase their level in the blood. And here again, how they might interact with a homeopathic and incompletely studied drug is not known.

The promise of the DOACs was that because of their wider therapeutic window, monitoring to assess the intensity of anticoagulation would not be necessary. While that has been the case, the bad news is that the manufacturers of the DOACs did not develop tests that could be used to determine just how anticoagulated a patient is when they come into the ER bleeding to death. Worse still, for the first several years they were available for prescription, no specific antidote had been developed. If Mr. McCabe had been on a DOAC that interacted with olive leaf extract like warfarin did, when he bled out of his penis, stopping the bleeding would have been a problem. Catastrophic bleeding with DOACs is a relatively rare event, but only because doctors can look at the label of whatever other prescription drugs patients are using to see if they increase or decrease DOAC levels. Olive leaf extract has no package insert with prescribing information. Its potential to interact with DOACs is as unknown as its interactions with warfarin.

Mr. McCabe survived and did well after his near-death experience. Thereafter, he took great pains to avoid unprescribed medications. Though admirable, it would not be an easy task in a world that relies on anti-inflammatories, analgesics, antihistamines, anti-diarrheals, antipyretics, antibiotics and a host of other commonly used medications available either over the counter or by prescription from healthcare professionals who have no idea if the drugs they prescribe or recommend are going to cause harm, directly or indirectly. Even when we know of potentially injurious drug interactions, like the risk of bleeding when ibuprofen is used with an anticoagulant, it is a daunting task to adequately inform all the patients who use drugs for common pain relief.

COMMENTARY

Congress passed legislation several decades ago to establish an agency to oversee the safety of food and drugs, the United States Food and Drug Administration. The new legislation held that all new drugs and medical devices would be required to demonstrate efficacy and safety by carrying out randomized and controlled clinical trials deemed by the new agency to be complete and accurate. In doing so, there would be assurance that the new therapies worked; also, each new product would carry a label clearly outlining exactly how effective it is and what its safety concerns are, so practicing doctors could have a detailed roadmap for its use.

Similarly, drugs that could be used without a prescription, that is, over the counter, would also have proof that they are effective for their indications, with precise instructions for their safe use. Many of the drugs that became available over the counter had transitioned from prescription use so there was a sufficient fund of knowledge about safety and efficacy before they were made available without a prescription.

But as we have seen in other stories, a gaping loophole in the regulations was that if a new product was considered a food derivative rather than a new drug, the pathway to marketing approval and oversight would be strikingly less stringent. Proof would still be needed that it did no harm, but that is not a particularly high hurdle. Unless someone is allergic, food derivatives, especially in small quantities, are unlikely to hurt healthy people. Elaborate studies of safety, like toxicology and animal testing, and normal volunteer experiments, would be a needless burden and were not mandated.

The big mistake was made on the efficacy side. In essence, the law said that to make a claim that a food-derived drug worked, testimony from anyone who took the product would suffice. If a nice elderly gentleman was willing to go on TV and say that capsules that were manufactured from jellyfish extract gave him "a memory like an elephant," the product could be marketed and advertised with a claim of improving mentation.

This lax requirement opened the floodgates for the development of a legion of products, advertised on TV and in print, that purport to treat and cure just about every symptom and disease known to mankind. The public was easily seduced into believing that food-derived substances were worth a try since they had no liability. The consequences, however, have been serious. First, patients frequently eschew the use of effective drugs for real indications in favor of homeopathy. Serious conditions like high blood pressure or diabetes may be undertreated or not treated at all in favor of supplements, with obvious repercussions. When given the choice between purchasing an expensive prescription drug with possible toxicity, and a celebrity-endorsed product advertised on television that has a somewhat lower price tag, most patients will choose the latter option. That is not to say that alternative medications are necessarily cheap. Depending on the indication and quantity, the cost may be as high or higher than that of prescription drugs, the full cost of the specious remedy borne by the patient with no insurance company contribution.

As we learned in the story of Mr. McCabe, alternative drugs have the potential to harm patients in several ways. St. John's Wort, for example, sold as a panacea for several common maladies, can alter the electrical stability of the heart, rendering the user susceptible to life-threatening cardiac arrhythmias. How many people have suffered a lethal heart arrhythmia while taking such an agent is impossible to know because there is no mechanism for reporting or cataloging serious adverse effects of alternative medications, as there is with prescription drugs.

Perhaps the most disappointing fallout from poor regulatory oversight of alternative medicine is the billions of dollars spent on ineffective remedies. Aggressive advertising is used in place of real science to convince the masses to buy and consume these products. And the obfuscation is intentional and clever. Listen carefully to the commercials in which a wise-sounding commentator says that "clinical studies have shown…" It wouldn't occur to most viewers to ask, "Which clinical studies?" Similarly, most people wouldn't suspect a person with an MD after their name of promoting a drug or device that has no worth. A doctor's willingness to provide testimony in a TV commercial must prove that the product they recommend is worthwhile, right? How such individuals can reconcile their feckless behavior with their Hippocratic Oath is a mystery. In any sane world, these individuals would have their medical licenses revoked. Our professional societies and licensing agents prefer to ignore their nefarious behavior. For years, Dr. Oz peddled worthless medicines on his television program and pocketed millions of dollars. Not only was he not censured by our profession, but he subsequently ran for political office and has now been put in charge of the largest medical insurance payer in the world, the Centers for Medicare and Medicaid Services.

Not to be forgotten are the purveyors of the idea that altering diet cures a multitude of diseases. Unquestionably, a carefully balanced diet has benefits, but fad diets fall flat every time and for a variety of reasons. First, the scientific rationale for drastic changes in dietary intake is poorly established. Most of the research consists of a few animal experiments with endpoints that make no sense for organisms that stand on two legs. Clinical research to support any of these diets is practically non-existent, and when present, usually consists of inadequately powered studies with non-relevant endpoints. Finally, fad diets are not sustainable because they are expensive and not palatable. Human beings will not continue to consume bad tasting food no matter the reputed benefit. One of my patients was pleased to tell me, "My new diet is simple. If the food tastes good, I spit it out."

The development of real and effective treatments for a disease that plagues millions is hard work. It requires billions of dollars and years of clinical trials, as we discussed in another story. It is human nature to seek out simple solutions to complex and possibly unsolvable problems. Alzheimer's disease is a prime example. Over the past few years, brilliant scientists have worked with pharmaceutical companies to develop treatments to prevent or remove deposits in the brain that are responsible for dementia. Despite some amazing progress, we are yet to come up with an affordable treatment that not only reduces the deposits but also improves mentation.

Alzheimer's is a horrible disease that we all want to avoid. Because conventional treatments are not available, many people look for alternatives. Enter the unprincipled purveyors of unproven therapies; all they need is enough money to advertise and a few people who believe their memory has improved. The elderly who don't want to accept that their mentation is slipping will pay premium prices to forestall the development of what is likely an inevitable, age-related decline. And when they take the product, they convince themselves that their memory and mentation are better.

The number of worthless treatments promoted for various maladies is legion. Their commonality is subjective, life-style improvement. Objectively measurable and important endpoints like freedom from stroke, heart attack, hospitalization, or death would be impossible to prove and thus are avoided by the snake oil salespeople. That doesn't mean that claims of extending life or avoiding serious vascular events are off the table. Chelation therapy is an example of a treatment that is supposed to clear the body of atherosclerosis, thus preventing heart attacks, despite no hard data to prove its efficacy.

Symptom improvement, on the other hand, is much more obtainable via a healthy dose of suggestibility and our old friend, the placebo effect. And if the claim is simply that you can "lead a better life" with vitamins or fish oil or olive leaf extract or stem cells, the potential for chicanery is inestimable. Mr. McCabe, our patient and a highly intelligent and sensitive man, felt better taking olive leaf extract, likely because he expected to feel better. What he didn't expect, and about which he was never warned, was blood gushing from his penis in the middle of the night.

CONCLUSION

Truly, the horse has left the barn. The multi-billion-dollar alternative medicine juggernaut is gathering momentum and will never be halted. Industry-supported lobbies are too strong, and legislators don't see why they need to interfere with a free enterprise that is generating taxable revenue without an obvious downside. Even if the laws were changed to improve oversight of alternative drugs, regulatory agencies don't have the bandwidth to take on this gargantuan task. And to add fuel to the fire, a new Secretary of Health and Human Services has been an ardent advocate of alternative medicines for serious diseases, intentionally ignoring or discounting hard scientific data of their worthlessness and showing blatant disregard of their potential hazards.

The fact is that people like the idea of taking something to improve their health. For decades, vitamins have been dispensed to children by worried parents. Recent data have proven beyond doubt that vitamins do nothing other than provide reassurance to parents that they are taking good care of their children. Do we therefore need to regulate once-a-day vitamins? As long as expectations are not excessive, the costs are not high and safety is assured, I believe not. However, it is important for patients and physicians to think through the alternative medicine concept in situations where vulnerable patients may be harmed. In this story, I have outlined some of the pitfalls of using substances about which little is known.

PATIENT ADVICE

Patients who are taking prescription drugs for serious indications, particularly those with a narrow therapeutic window, like antiarrhythmic, anticonvulsant or anticoagulant medications, need to be circumspect when considering an alternative medication. Likewise, physicians should dissuade patients from using supplements if there is insufficient knowledge regarding how they are metabolized and excreted. As with direct-to-consumer advertising for prescription drugs, cautions should be incorporated along with product label warnings to avoid a catastrophe. It needs to be clear that these remedies have not been proven to treat or cure any disease, and the disclaimer prominently displayed, not relegated to small print at the bottom of the screen.

Similarly, advice from a doctor on television who emphasizes that he or she is a "board certified expert" needs to be carefully considered. If a professional requires a commercial to convince the public that something is "good medicine," chances are that mainstream medicine and good science are not in agreement, and that there is no certainty of benefit. Consumers should lobby governmental officials to prohibit advertisements that have no good scientific basis and to dissuade bureaucrats with no medical training to advocate for worthless treatments. After all, the whole reason we have regulatory agencies is to ensure best treatments—isn't it?

Story 10: Physician Burnout is Real and Really Bad for Everyone

"The hours are terrible, the pay is terrible, you're underappreciated, disrespected and frequently physically endangered. But there's no better job in the world." —Joseph Lister

NARRATIVE

Mr. Han was a 45-year-old Asian man, an American success story. He came to a small town in Ohio from Korea with his parents when he was ten, joining an extended Korean family who had established a beachhead there. He and his parents spoke little English, but at their insistence, he and his siblings graduated from high school. Mr. Han went on to a vocational school where he learned how to be a carpenter, and over the next several years, he was steadily employed in construction jobs. He and his wife lived in a pleasant rural neighborhood, where they raised a son and daughter. As a member of the carpenters' union, he had good health insurance. This was important to Mr. Han because both of his parents had suffered from diabetes and high blood pressure and had died in their sixties. Mr. Han, who had inherited the same diseases, was determined to maintain his good health, to be around for his family.

To that end, Mr. Han sought out an excellent primary care doctor near his home. Dr. Robb had a stellar reputation in the community because she spent time with each of her patients and managed them carefully. Over the fifteen years that Mr. and Mrs. Han had been her patients, they had developed an excellent relationship. Mr. Han was compliant with the medications that Dr. Robb prescribed to lower his blood pressure and manage his diabetes, and both diseases were well controlled. Mr. Han was comfortable discussing all his medical problems and drug side effects, including the sensitive issue of erectile dysfunction, which Dr. Robb had treated successfully with the elimination of a beta-blocker that was being used to lower his blood pressure. Mr.

Han and his wife truly believed that their good health was a direct result of their close liaison with Dr. Robb and her office staff, and that without them, they would be lost.

All was well until Mrs. Han greeted Mr. Han, upon his return from a hard day's work, with a sad face. They had received a letter from Dr. Robb's office informing them that she had decided to switch to a "concierge" practice at the end of the calendar year. Mr. Han had heard about such things but knew little about them. The letter provided some explanation, but Mr. Han had an appointment with Dr. Robb the following month. He was anxious to find out what was happening and what he might do to keep seeing her.

As usual, Dr. Robb began Mr. Han's appointment with a thorough interview and physical examination, followed by review and renewal of his medications. This didn't take long because Mr. Han felt well and had no new complaints. When he asked about her plans, she told Mr. Han how sorry she was to have to change her practice. She explained that she had become overwhelmed by the effort needed to take excellent care of her patients. She was putting in long hours and was unhappy. Her life at home had suffered significantly, and she simply couldn't continue to be away from her children and her husband as much as she had been in the past few years.

On the bright side, Dr. Robb hoped that Mr. and Mrs. Han would be able to stay with her. There would be several advantages to doing so, including longer visit times, better staffing at the office, and full access via cell phone or email. They could contact her at any time with questions. Unfortunately, becoming one of her "clients" was going to cost $3000 per year for Mr. Han and $5000 per year if he wanted to include his wife. She explained this was an access fee and Mr. Han would continue to have co-pays and other out-of-pocket expenses. Her "concierge" service was an extra charge on top of what she billed their insurance company for her medical services.

Mr. Han understood Dr. Robb's predicament but was insistent. Why couldn't he stay on with her as a regular patient? Dr. Robb explained that caring for her "special" patients would require all her time. The company that had recruited her and was financing her new practice demanded that she limit her patient load to the first four hundred who signed up, pared down from the almost three thousand patients she currently had in her practice.

Mr. Han told Dr. Robb that he would have to discuss the issue with his wife, but that the extra $5000 per year would be difficult for their already stretched budget to absorb. Dr. Robb said she understood. If they couldn't sign up, she would try to help Mr. Han find a new primary care doctor nearby.

Mr. and Mrs. Han's discussion about signing up for Dr. Robb's concierge practice was a sad and brief one. They agreed it was simply not possible to spend that much money on a medical care luxury. Besides, Dr. Robb had done such a great job of preserving their good health that they rarely called her for emergencies or even for urgencies. They didn't need more frequent or prolonged appointments. They were both relatively young, and the situation was unlikely to change anytime soon.

Reluctantly, they declined to join Dr. Robb's panel of patients and began the hunt for a new primary care doctor. They didn't think the search was going to be easy, but they never anticipated just how difficult it would be. The population of their small town had grown much faster than the supply of doctors had. Also, many of the best doctors in general practice had decided to "go concierge" like Dr. Robb, and those who hadn't were no longer open for new patients.

Mr. Han was in a panic. It was only with Dr. Robb's intercession that he was able to get an appointment for himself and his wife with a new primary care practice, but six months hence. Dr. Robb was kind enough to make sure they had enough medication to get them through to that appointment, and fortunately they stayed healthy in the interim.

Mr. Han's first appointment at the new practice was a shock. He arrived on time but had to wait an hour to be admitted to an examination room and another half-hour until a practitioner arrived. It wasn't the doctor he had signed up to see, but rather a nurse practitioner who was in a rush. She asked a few questions about Mr. Han's health, performed a rudimentary physical examination, reviewed his medications and renewed them with his pharmacy, all within about five minutes. Standing at the computer table with her back to Mr. Han, she typed away while she asked if he had any questions. Mr. Han told her he couldn't think of any, which seemed to be the response the nurse practitioner was hoping for. She quickly logged off the computer, told Mr. Han to return in about six months and to call if he had any problems in the interim. And she was gone.

A few days later, his wife had the same experience. She didn't have an opportunity to meet the new doctor or to have a significant interaction with the nurse practitioner, who saw her briefly. Mr. and Mrs. Han were distressed, feeling disconnected from the healthcare providers now responsible for their care.

Over the next several months, things didn't go well for the Hans. On the few occasions they called the practice, it took days to get a response and then it came not from a doctor but from one of the nurses who rushed through the conversation and didn't answer their questions completely. Mr. and Mrs. Han didn't feel motivated to maintain their diet and exercise programs. They had little confidence that they could expect good medical care when they needed it. They felt like a numbered commodity without the sustaining therapeutic relationship they had enjoyed with Dr. Robb for so many years.

Predictably, Mr. and Mrs. Han fell off the wagon. By not taking good care of themselves, their excellent medical condition deteriorated. Without a firm guiding hand, Mr. Han struggled with his blood pressure and blood sugar control, and Mrs. Han's weight ballooned as her dietary guidance disappeared and her questions went unanswered. It would only be a matter of time until they would suffer a healthcare crisis and end up in an emergency room or worse.

CASE EXPLANATION

What happened to Dr. Robb is unfortunately all too common. She was dedicated to her patients and spent abundant time with each of them, carefully managing their illnesses and risk factors, doing whatever was necessary to maintain their good health. Unfortunately, she did so at a significant cost to herself and her family that she couldn't sustain. She was crushed by her job. Not only did she have to manage her patients, but she also had to participate in the business of her medical practice, the complexity of which had become staggering.

For all her hard work, Dr. Robb was paid poorly. Like most physicians, she was not compensated for the extra time she spent answering patient phone calls and messages, or for the charting she needed to do in the evenings and on weekends to keep up with her workload. She spent enormous amounts of her own time writing letters and filling out forms so that her patients could get special services like handicap parking. The healthcare system that employed her mandated the number of patients she was expected to see per day. She was allotted ten minutes for each established patient and twenty for a new patient, but her visits almost always went overtime. Everyone, including her employer, knew that the visit times were absurdly short, but they insisted that she maintain a high patient volume to optimize revenue.

As a result, Dr. Robb had to rush to see all her patients to keep the waiting room from overflowing and to finish all her appointments before the office closed. During the day, there was no time to take a break, let alone write notes or answer phone calls. Any clerical work, including patient notes, had to be done in her supposed "free time." The strain on Dr. Robb carried over into her private life. Her husband, a patient man with a job of his own, tried not to harry her but was disappointed with the direction their married life was taking. With family time shrinking, he had to assume almost all the childcare responsibility and house chores while his wife labored at the computer in their den every evening. It was not a sustainable situation.

Because of time pressure, Dr. Robb was petrified that by hurrying through her patient schedule, she would miss something important. Remember that as a primary care physician, Dr. Robb was responsible for all aspects of the patient's care. She could and did refer to specialists, when necessary, but her salary was contingent on limiting the number of referrals. She was provided with a list of consultants and how much each of them spent on tests. To save money for the practice, she was discouraged from referring to consultants at the high end of testing costs, regardless of how skilled that person might be.

To make an appropriate referral, Dr. Robb had to at least begin to understand the patient's problem and initiate diagnostic testing and treatment. All of that would take time she simply didn't have in her practice. What Dr. Robb feared the most was getting sued for malpractice, a trauma discussed in a previous story. And the risk of that happening was multiplying in the pressure cooker that was her everyday practice.

The solution for thousands of good primary care doctors like Dr. Robb is to turn to private equity companies to set them up in a "concierge practice." The patient cost to join such a practice varies around the country but ranges from $2000 to $5000 per patient. For the affluent elderly, with a host of medical problems, the investment makes sense. And there are more than enough such patients who want to enroll in a concierge practice to make it a seller's market.

Those patients who were able to stay with Dr. Robb would be pleased with their situation, as well they should. Not only would they be able to spend more time with a highly competent and compassionate doctor, but she would visit them in the hospital and be an ombudsman for them during their acute illnesses. And texts or calls with questions would be answered promptly and with kind understanding.

However, the consequence of a care upheaval like this one is that a very large number of unfortunate patients like Mr. and Mrs. Han are cast adrift into an environment where there are simply not enough primary care doctors to go around.

Mr. and Mrs. Han were lucky to find a replacement primary care practice, but, as with so many practices that have survived, this one was staffed mainly with nurse practitioners or physician assistants. It is estimated that nearly half of primary care practitioners in the United States are non-physicians and the percentage is expected to increase exponentially. At each visit, the Hans were seen by a new person, so it would never be possible for them to establish a therapeutic relationship like the one they enjoyed with Dr. Robb. How important that liaison was could only be appreciated until it was gone. Mr. and Mrs. Han's health status deteriorated, not rapidly but insidiously and inevitably. Tests would no longer be used to confirm diagnoses but used as a substitute for a good history and physical examination, which their new practitioners didn't value. Not only did the physician extenders have inadequate time to do a proper job, but they had never been trained to be excellent bedside clinicians. They were robots who followed algorithms to determine which tests to order and which drugs and treatments to prescribe. They spent most of the visit clacking away at the computer, their backs turned to their patients. Lacking a deep understanding of the diseases they were treating necessarily limited their ability to give insightful answers to questions. A true therapeutic relationship in which questions could be asked and answered with confidence was impossible.

COMMENTARY

Delivering the highest quality medical care is hard work. It is time consuming, energy draining, and lifestyle corroding. In years gone by, people who pursued the medical profession understood this and were willing to make a significant personal sacrifice because they viewed medicine as a calling. And when they worked hard, they were doing sacred work, helping patients through difficult illnesses, and reaping the reward of seeing those patients heal and return to normal function. They were treated well by their community and by their patients, having earned their respect. They didn't make a fortune, but they were paid well. One old-time doctor told me that his patients expected him to drive a nice car, because that meant he was successful. He drove a Buick, a high-end automobile back then. But he deliberately didn't drive a Cadillac because he worried that his patients would think he was making too much money and profiting from their suffering.

Modern medicine is an entirely different animal. No longer is any premium placed on being a good bedside clinician. Talking to and examining patients is not rewarded in the same way that our system pays for procedures and tests. Medical students are seduced by technology and are drawn toward specialties that will allow them to spend copious amounts of time in operating suites and procedure rooms. When they graduate, they seek jobs that generate great streams of revenue and are rewarded by their employers with large salaries, a prerequisite for paying down the oppressive debt that the medical education system foisted on them.

The dearth of primary care physicians is not difficult to understand. Medical students are not incentivized to pursue primary care as a specialty for many reasons. They spend almost no time in a general medicine environment during their training. In fact, the outpatient experience during their residencies is woefully inadequate.

Primary care physicians are expected to know a lot about many different diseases and when they can't keep up, they become triage agents who send patients to various specialists for second-level care. They look for short-cuts to get through their ridiculously packed calendars, like throwing antibiotics at just about everyone who may have an infection when they just don't have the time to do a thorough examination. What this profligate prescription policy has spawned is the emergence of killer bacteria, resistant to just about all antibiotics. Primary care doctors carry out few procedures that generate revenue and their salaries thus are absurdly low. This is a particular handicap for young doctors who complete their training hundreds of thousands of dollars in debt. What primary care doctors do for their patients is simply not valued by bean-counting administrators whose only metric is revenue generation.

What can be done to increase the supply of primary care doctors? There are several obvious solutions. Our legislators thought that simply increasing the number of medical schools and graduating more medical students would solve the problem, but it has not. Newly minted doctors have the same incentives to seek out lucrative specialties as their predecessors, so the net result has been an increase in the number of specialists. Expanding the number of medical school slots while scaring bright young people away from medicine has had the effect of significantly diluting the quality of medical school graduates. For example, we have seen a disturbing increase in the number of students who fail their board examinations on their first attempt.

Loan forgiveness is now being used as an incentive for young doctors to enter general practice, especially in underserved areas of the country. This has worked to some extent, but medical students who could take advantage of this opportunity are asked to make an early career decision about a specialty based on financial need. Most would rather train in a more attractive specialty like ophthalmology or plastic surgery and receive a bigger salary to more quicky pay off their debt. This is especially true for the growing number of trainees who marry in medical school and need to consider their spouses' careers when deciding about their own practice location.

A few elite medical schools have done away with medical school tuition altogether, eliminating or significantly reducing the crushing debt graduating doctors face. This decision was made possible by high profile philanthropic gifts earmarked specifically for that purpose. Free tuition for medical students, especially if it is tied to a post-graduate service responsibility, will have an enormous impact on our doctor shortage.

Easing the financial burden on graduating doctors is not a pipe dream. Many medical schools have seen their endowments skyrocket through high returns on long-term investment portfolios and, even more importantly, from royalties paid on institutional patents that led to breakthrough treatments. A prominent example is the academic research that brought COVID-19 vaccines to market during the pandemic. But despite these windfalls, almost all medical schools have only raised their tuition, using their reserves to put up more buildings and to reward their executives with higher salaries, all the while preserving their tax-exempt status as "nonprofit" institutions. Sharp reductions in federal subsidies and grants to medical schools, carried out by the present administration, will undoubtedly lead to even higher tuitions and fees for young people brave enough to seek a medical degree.

Adding doctors who have been trained in other countries could also help address the shortage of primary care physicians. However, our medical boards continue to make it difficult for foreign medical graduates to get US jobs. In most states, well-trained physicians are required to complete residency training in a certified US program before they can be fully licensed to practice. Asking a fully boarded internist or consultant from the UK to repeat internship and residency here is preposterous, a remnant of political pressure brought to bear by US professional organizations to preserve the job market for US graduates. Well-trained Ukrainian and Afghani doctors who escaped their countries are unable to work as physicians even though most of them are more competent than the wet-behind-the-ears American graduates who turn up their noses at primary care.

The solution for many practices is physician extenders. Supervision is the fundamental issue in training such people to close the care gap. As illustrated in this story, Mr. and Mrs. Han signed up for a primary care practice but never saw the doctor who was circulating somewhere in the office. It was never made clear to them whether the nurse practitioner who saw them was supervised. This caused them significant anxiety. They were afraid to ask the nurse practitioner if the doctor approved of her decisions, so they accepted what she said, hoping that a doctor was somehow in control.

For whatever reason it occurs, including a dearth of primary care doctors, physician burnout is a major problem, and it is not being adequately addressed. Doctors commit suicide and suffer serious mental health issues at a rate much higher than that of the general population. Over half of doctors in practice admit to having anxiety and depression related to their work. The most frightening part is that they frequently ignore their symptoms and try to soldier through. They may self-medicate or, in the worst cases, resort to drugs and alcohol, but for all of them, their mental health problems have a negative impact on their job performance. It is simply unreasonable to expect a highly distracted and depressed physician to deliver consistent, compassionate, and skilled care.

When asked what has led to their burnout, physicians are quick to start with the electronic medical record, a topic covered elsewhere in this book. Comprehensive documentation of every aspect of a patient's care is an overwhelming and unnecessary burden that has not been lifted or modified. They also list the barrage of messages they must respond to throughout their workday, and the fear that they will miss or ignore a complaint that will lead to a catastrophe. Consider the impact of new laws in several states that allow patients to access their laboratory reports immediately, even before their physicians have had time to review them. What has resulted is an exponential increase in the number of anxious patients calling physician offices with worries caused by their inability to interpret test results and decipher their clinical significance.

The naïve will argue that artificial intelligence (AI) is the answer to clinician burnout. While AI may provide some help, it will also place physicians and patients in jeopardy. If not carefully supervised, an undetected AI mistake will be the practitioner's responsibility. With many arguing for AI autonomy for many tasks such as drug prescribing, if and how doctors and other healthcare providers will oversee AI is not at all clear, but proper supervision will likely add significantly to the practitioner's burden.

Keeping up with the medical literature is a nearly impossible task for physicians, as is attending conferences to ensure that they have enough continuing education credits to maintain licensure. They are also expected to comply with a bewildering array of regulatory requirements and paperwork in the name of "compliance." Every year, a large batch of computer modules are dumped on them so they can document that they know what to do when they observe a violent patient or an active shooter. Never mind that the subject matter doesn't change; it still takes as long to go through the material no matter how redundant or irrelevant to one's practice.

As an example, consider that physicians who want a license to dispense controlled substances (including something as mundane as sleeping pills) must now complete eight hours of computer-based instruction that has little to no bearing on their practice. How about compelling doctors who never see children to complete several hours of training in how to recognize child abuse before they can be licensed? Or the imposition of courses and examinations to recertify and then maintain certification in every medical specialty, and the many hours these exercises consume in the already hectic life of the physician. Take the physician who attained board status in Internal Medicine, General Cardiology and then Cardiac Electrophysiology. Recertifying for each of these every ten years places that person on an endless merry-go-round of self-study and examinations that consumes hours of what would otherwise be family or personal time. And the punchline: in the few instances in which the value of these extra requirements has been intensively studied, they have never been shown to improve patient outcomes or patient satisfaction.

It should therefore not be surprising that doctors are constantly looking for a way out. Dr. Robb decided to go "concierge." Others abandon patient care and take jobs in industry or government. Some quit medicine entirely and become carpenters or plumbers, where they won't necessarily get an increase in their compensation but will certainly improve their quality of life. At a recent alumni luncheon, I reunited with an internist who left practice years ago. I remembered him as a frustrated and hostile individual, but the smile on his face at our meeting was unmistakable. He had decided to pursue his love of woodworking and was delighted to have been present for his children's activities.

But the largest contributor to the physician shortage is early retirement. This is particularly disturbing since over one-third of active physicians in the US are at an age when retirement is feasible, especially in the present economic environment when retirement accounts are robust enough to support a reasonable lifestyle for their remaining years.

Interestingly, many if not most physicians who retire early from full-time practice are highly amenable to practicing part-time. This could be a great source of physicians, particularly those under the age of 75 who are in their prime as clinicians, to work in economically depressed areas. But our broken system fails us again, imposing exorbitant costs for malpractice insurance and office overhead making part-time employment unworkable for most.

Many physicians, particularly those in academic medicine, have eased the burden of practice by participating in clinical research and teaching. Most of the important clinical trials are funded by industry, and physicians have been compensated for their time performing the research, aiding in the exploration of new therapies and instructing their peers when new treatments become generally available. Although there have been a few abuses, the overwhelming majority of this activity is not only aboveboard but essential for success in the development of better medicines, devices and procedures.

But the federal government has chosen to make public how much money is paid by industry to specific doctors, on the unproven assumption doing so will have a positive impact on the quality of research and patient attitudes about their physicians. As discussed in another story, hundreds of millions of dollars have been spent on the "Open Payments" program, which so far has had no impact on the money paid to doctors who work with industry or on the quality or quantity of studies that are completed through physician-industry collaboration. All it has done is impose another administrative burden on doctors and create the impression of wrongdoing, further lowering physician self-esteem and sowing the seed of mistrust in the very few patients who pay any attention to those data.

Our legislators further burden doctors by passing laws that not only make no sense, but also place doctors in direct jeopardy. Argue what you will about the morality of anti-abortion laws, but when doctors are threatened with criminal prosecution for caring for their patients in the best way they know how, the consequences are enormous. Such laws intimidate young doctors and doctors-in-training either to completely abandon specialties like obstetrics and gynecology, or to emigrate from states that foolishly pass misguided legislation. The result is a gross undersupply of competent physicians in large regions of the country, transforming childbirth, a usually happy occasion, into a scary and sometimes dangerous proposition.

CONCLUSION

When asked if they would once again pursue a career in medicine, a disturbing percentage of doctors say no, and do so sadly but emphatically. Even worse, these disgruntled people counsel their children and other bright young people to avoid the medical profession. Asked why, they shake their heads and reply that the work is just too hard and that they feel undervalued. While they were willing to make personal sacrifices during their training, they expected much more from their years in practice. Those of us who became physicians decades ago know how wonderful our profession was back then, and how well we could balance work and our private lives. We also know that those who dare to go to medical school today will not have the same perception of medicine as a profession. For them, it will be a punch-the-clock shift job, more or less.

Can we somehow rescue physicians and restore our profession? To do so would take a monumental and coordinated effort by government, hospital administration, and our professional organizations. We can begin by lightening the load, to lift many of the burdens off the doctors' shoulders. Obvious fixes include scribes to help with the EMR, longer appointment time slots, fewer needless compliance courses, tort reform to lessen the fear of malpractice lawsuits, and more help from supervised physician extenders and office staff. An enlightened legislature that doesn't presume to practice medicine would also be a boon.

But most fundamental to a solution is healthcare leadership that is truly committed to doctor well-being. The suits who run healthcare systems are not motivated in any way to do this, and neither are legislators who have no understanding of medicine and are not interested in listening to people who do. Despite collecting our dues and continuous requests for donations for political action committees, professional medical associations have done a dreadful job of representing physician interests at a governmental level, allowing laws and regulations to be enacted that place doctors under enormous pressure. And for what? Despite paying lip service to evidence-based medicine, not one of medicine's overseers has taken the time to prove that the time sinks imposed on doctors make one iota of difference in patient outcomes.

We need doctors with practice experience to represent us, and we need our informed patients to be our advocates. And if job actions are necessary to get the public's attention, sympathy and cooperation, so be it.

PATIENT ADVICE

It is difficult to overstate the benefits of having a great doctor—and a great doctor is hard to find. A good place to start looking is your own community. Ask respected friends, colleagues, and family members about their primary care physicians. Learn who works in your network, research their reputations, and try to meet with them in person.

A successful search carries great dividends. Patients who have confidence in their doctors not only have fewer health crises, but also have better outcomes from common diseases, across the board. Maintaining those individuals who have the courage to train and practice as exemplary physicians is vital to the health of our medical care system. It is a simple and well-proven fact that patients have better outcomes when they are treated by an unburdened physician.

Unfortunately, a band-aid will not close a gaping wound. Either we all act quickly to repair what is causing doctors to burn out, or we accept an inevitable decline in the quality of care. Advocating for legislation to increase the supply of well-trained healthcare providers and proper allocation of the billions of dollars spent on medical care in the US will help stem the tide. How far quality will plunge, while legislators and professional leaders turn a blind eye to this evolving crisis and pretend that all is well is anybody's guess. But no one pretends to have seen the bottom of that well.

Story 11: It's All About the Money: For-Profit Outpatient Procedural Centers

"God heals and the doctor takes the fees." —Benjamin Franklin

NARRATIVE

Ms. Nell was a young Caucasian woman, an only child who had suffered through a troubled adolescence. She loved her parents but resented them for having passed along genes that predisposed her to acne, asthma and, even worse, being overweight. The asthma was controlled. Although she had flares that required emergency room visits during childhood, she had been attack-free for several years. The steroids she had taken intermittently had exacerbated her weight gain, given her more pimples, and made her generally miserable.

According to her medical records, Ms. Nell battled her weight problem mightily, starting as soon as she became aware of how difficult life could be for a "fat person." In her pre-treatment interviews, Ms. Nell explained to her doctor that she was regularly bullied and shamed at school by the "in crowd" who thought fat jokes were funny. Ms. Nell had almost no friends, and those she hung out with had the same weight problem she did. She was never asked out on a real date, and the only boys who showed any interest had their own weight problems or were so socially awkward that she was uncomfortable being around them.

Her parents were sensitive to the issues and, with her pediatrician, helped her try just about everything to lose weight including various diets, medications, behavioral therapy, and even a stint at a "fat farm" that didn't go well at all.

When Ms. Nell graduated from high school, she was not interested in going off to college. She settled for a job behind the counter at the local Starbucks while continuing to live with her parents. To preserve a modicum of ego, she told her family and her few friends that she would soon begin night classes at the local community college.

However, it turned out that regular employment agreed with Ms. Nell. Getting out of bed early and working every day motivated her to take better care of herself. Instead of going directly home from work and snacking, Ms. Nell made it a habit to stop at the local Y for an exercise session. She met a few like-minded souls there, and their friendship kept her visits regular and meaningful. The group would regularly go to dinner together after their exercise, careful to select places that served nutritious food in modest quantities. She told her physician that they laughed with the waiter when offered dessert and reveled in finishing off their meal with a low-calorie espresso.

To help her accelerate her weight loss, Ms. Nell's primary care doctor recommended a prescription for one of the new injectable drugs that Ms. Nell was able to purchase at a reasonable price, thanks to the good health insurance her employer provided. With medication, diet, and exercise, Ms. Nell lost thirty pounds over the next year, and her progress led to a major improvement in her self-esteem.

Ms. Nell's parents were excited to see their daughter's positive life change and promised to do whatever they could to maintain the momentum. So, when she announced at dinner that she was interested in having a liposuction procedure, they were receptive, albeit skeptical. She explained that despite her weight loss, she had retained a mass of adipose tissue over her abdomen and hips that would likely not resolve. Fully clothed and with support underwear, she had been able to mask the protuberances, but with summer coming she was afraid she would not look good in a bathing suit, even a one-piece.

Ms. Nell had researched the issue and was sure that the best solution was to have the fat tissue literally vacuumed out. Liposuction was common and available at several places in her area. She had seen an advertisement on the internet for a cosmetic surgery center not far from where she lived. The center offered the procedure at a reasonable price. Cost was Ms. Nell's principal concern since her insurance company considered liposuction a cosmetic procedure without a health benefit and therefore would not pay for it. The insurance company ignored her doctor's records that carefully documented the psychological problems that Ms. Nell had suffered because of her weight.

They also refused to read the articles her doctor provided pointing out that the procedure produced tangible psychological improvement, less depression and need for psychotropic drugs and counseling, and less suicidality, a known and common complication of body shaming.

With the insurance company's firm rejection, the $4,000 that the procedure would cost would have to be paid out-of-pocket. Ms. Nell asked her parents if they could float her a loan so she could have the procedure soon, without having to wait until she saved enough money out of her modest salary. They agreed.

Ms. Nell scheduled an appointment with the center and was assigned to Dr. Bank, a newly minted plastic surgeon who now performed procedures at the center. She immediately liked Dr. Bank. Not only was he relatively young and handsome, but he was kind. He examined Ms. Nell carefully and then sat with her for several minutes to explain the procedure and answer her questions. He told her that the consent form she would sign would list several potential adverse effects, including death, but given her good health he expected the procedure to go well with a minimal chance for harm and a high likelihood of a rapid recovery.

Ms. Nell was surprised and excited that Dr. Bank would be able to perform her procedure the following week; her parents and she had anticipated a longer wait. As instructed, she arrived at the center at 7 a.m. accompanied by her mother who would wait on site and drive her home after recovery from anesthesia.

She was greeted by a friendly nurse who asked her to change into a gown before being loaded onto a stretcher and parked in the pre-operative area. There, Ms. Nell was the center of attention; there were no other waiting patients. Her nurse took her vital signs, started an intravenous line, placed some electrodes on her chest to monitor her heart rate and rhythm, and attached a finger clip to measure the amount of oxygen in her blood. The nurse also went through a checklist including assurance that Ms. Nell had had nothing to eat or drink after the preceding midnight.

The nurse was followed by an anesthesiologist who asked a few questions, listened to her heart and lungs with his stethoscope, and pronounced everything to be in good order. Ms. Nell asked the anesthesiologist if her history of asthma would be an issue. He reassured her that he would be able to treat an airway problem if one arose. Since they were not planning general anesthesia, but only conscious sedation, her asthma would not be a factor. He promised she would be relaxed and comfortable throughout the procedure.

Minutes later, Ms. Nell was wheeled into the procedure room where Dr. Bank greeted her cheerfully, again reassuring her that the procedure would be fast and easy. He noted that she would have some pain and bruising for a few days after the operation but it would be managed with ice packs and an oral analgesic.

The anesthesiologist repeated her vital signs and then used her IV to administer Versed and fentanyl in relatively small doses, just enough to induce sleep. He then nodded to Dr. Bank that he could proceed with the liposuction procedure.

Ms. Nell's history, the pre-operation procedures, and what happened in the operating room and then over the ensuing thirty minutes would be detailed in office records, affidavits, depositions, and trial testimony by Dr. Bank, the anesthesiologist, and the nurse who assisted with the procedure. By all accounts, the liposuction procedure was carried out without incident. Dr. Bank was able to extract several grams of fat tissue from a few punctures over the lateral abdomen, exactly as he had intended. Ms. Nell's vital signs, including her heart rate, respiratory rate and blood pressure, remained stable. The anesthesiologist administered only a bit more "happy juice" to keep her asleep and restful. Dr. Bank finished the procedure in short order, and Ms. Nell was prepared for transfer to the recovery area.

During the stretcher ride, things started falling apart. Very suddenly, Ms. Nell started having trouble breathing. She gasped for air and had a sharp drop in her blood oxygen saturation. Aware of her asthma history, the anesthesiologist hurried her into the recovery area, ordered epinephrine and a bronchodilator, and attached a nasal cannula to deliver oxygen. With these measures, Ms. Nell seemed to stabilize. Though still not fully awake, her breathing was less strident, and her oxygenation improved, albeit not back to normal.

Dr. Bank was summoned to the recovery area and was relieved to see Ms. Nell's improvement. He asked the anesthesiologist if she might require transfer to a local hospital emergency room. The anesthesiologist advised waiting a bit longer to see how Ms. Nell felt when she was fully awake. Dr. Bank agreed. The anesthesiologist cautioned that transferring patients emergently after a routine procedure was not good publicity for their surgical center and

Dr. Bank had only recently started practicing at this facility.

The plaintiff's attorneys would later argue that this delay in transfer was a critical factor in determining Ms. Nell's ultimate outcome. Because thirty minutes later, Ms. Nell, now mostly awake, again complained of an inability to breathe. This was accompanied by a sharp drop in the oxygen in her system as well as a fall in her heart rate and blood pressure. The anesthesiologist, who had been seeing another patient, hurried to the bedside to observe Ms. Nell turn blue and start seizing. He called for an intubation tray and, despite her seizure activity, was able to insert an endotracheal tube in seconds. However, ventilating her using an Ambu bag and 100% oxygen didn't make a difference. Ms. Nell's status didn't improve. She remained hypoxic and hypotensive.

The staff called for an ambulance, which arrived in about ten minutes. The crew arrived at a full code situation. Nurses were performing CPR while Dr. Bank administered emergency medication. The ambulance crew was experienced and knew that a transfer during resuscitation would be difficult. CPR had to be interrupted several times during the process, but they managed to get Ms. Nell out of the center and into the ambulance within another ten minutes.

Ms. Nell's mother was frantic. She had heard the sirens and feared that something had happened to her daughter, but it wasn't until Dr. Bank came out of the restricted area and into the waiting room that she was fully briefed. She was told that her daughter was "stable" and being transferred to the local hospital, only a few miles away. If she felt up to it, it would be a good idea for her to drive there herself to help with her daughter's admission. Dr. Bank promised to meet them at the emergency room.

As it turned out, a hospital admission didn't happen. On arrival in the ER, resuscitation continued but it was obviously not working. Ms. Nell had no blood pressure or heart rhythm. The doctors administered multiple drugs in an attempt to start her heart and raise her blood pressure, to no avail. The community hospital had no facilities to place her on extracorporeal support, and the ER staff knew that she would not endure another transfer to a facility with a heart-lung machine. Though it was obvious at this point that Ms. Nell would not survive, the ER physician requested that resuscitation continue until he had a chance to ask the parents if they would consent to organ donation.

Ms. Nell's mother arrived at the ER around the same time and was joined by her husband whom she had called in transit. They waited anxiously for some word from the ER staff. Dr. Bank arrived soon thereafter and tried to reassure them that their daughter was in good hands and that everything was being done. When asked what had happened, he said their daughter likely had a severe asthma attack that had closed off her airway and made it impossible for her to get sufficient oxygen. The anesthesiologist quickly administered the correct reversal agents, and she had improved, but then she deteriorated again and became unresponsive. He told them how sorry he was.

When the ER doctor emerged a few minutes later to inform Mr. and Mrs. Nell that their daughter would not recover, they collapsed into each other's arms and cried hysterically. It took several minutes for them to compose themselves enough to address the urgent question the ER doctor had asked: would they consent to organ donation? Ms. Nell's father who worked in the pharmaceutical industry told the ER doctor that he was sympathetic to the idea and that his daughter had signed an organ donation card when she got her driver's license. But he also wanted his daughter to have an autopsy. To help his wife and him heal, they simply had to know why their daughter had died. They were nonplussed that asthma was the cause since it had been so long since her last acute attack.

The ER doctor informed the organ procurement bureau that during organ extraction there would need to be an examination of the body to determine the cause of death. The agency assured him that identifying the cause of death was an important part of their job because it would determine the viability of any organs they harvested. Ms. Nell remained on the ventilator with active chest compressions while she was taken to the operating room where organ extraction was completed. She was pronounced dead, and her body was handed over to the hospital pathologist for an unnecessary formal autopsy. Everyone in the operating room knew exactly why Ms. Nell had died.

CASE EXPLANATION
Ms. Nell was a healthy young woman who died from a complication of cosmetic surgery. Such deaths and serious complications from plastic surgery are fortunately uncommon but they are not rare—and when they do occur, it can be a full-blown catastrophe. The idea that a young person lost her life to look better in a bathing suit might seem absurd, but all surgery carries

risk, and some of that hazard can be mortal. That's why death is listed on the patient consent form, though usually glossed over by the surgeon, just as it was in this case.

What happened to Ms. Nell? Fortunately, her parents consented to organ donation and a postmortem examination without which the cause of death would never have been discovered, and presumed to be an asthma attack. Ms. Nell died of a fat embolism, a known complication of liposuction. In essence, during the procedure, Dr. Bank had inadvertently transected a large vein with the trocar he was using to suck out adipose tissue. When he withdrew the vacuum device, a large chunk of fat that remained in its lumen entered the vein and traveled to the right side of the heart and thence into the pulmonary arteries. The blockage it caused in those arteries prevented oxygenation of the blood. With severe deoxygenation, the heart could not function normally, nor could the brain and other vital organs. The only treatment that could have saved Ms. Nell's life was operative removal of the fat embolus or emboli if multiple, but that wouldn't have been possible without circulatory support. All those measures would have had to be implemented within minutes and at a center with advanced catheterization capabilities.

Not surprisingly, Mr. and Mrs. Nell sued Dr. Bank and the outpatient surgery center for wrongful death. The case was settled for a few million dollars, effectively closed the center, sent Dr. Bank off to pursue his craft in another state, and enriched the plaintiff malpractice attorney who didn't have to work hard to win the case and collect 40 percent of the award.

The investigation carried out by the plaintiff and defense attorneys brought to light several important facts about the case, many of which were included in the narrative. The handsome Dr. Bank was nefarious. He had been sued previously for operative complications and denied staff privileges at several area hospitals, which is why he was working at a free-standing surgical center. Part of his incompetence could be blamed not only on shoddy training, but also on a marked lack of experience. During discovery, he admitted to having performed fewer than 100 liposuction procedures since completing his training, with "a couple of complications." As a result, Dr. Bank had few referrals, which explained why the surgical center's waiting area was nearly empty on the day he was operating there.

Because of her youth and the low-risk procedure, Ms. Nell didn't need a costly and elaborate pre-operative screening. But she also had not had a complete history and physical examination by the anesthesiologist or by the surgeon. Had that occurred, the issue of her asthma might have been clarified. The truth was that her asthma issue was quiescent. As frequently happened with children, she had mostly outgrown her airway susceptibility. So, when she had her initial decompensation, time would not have been wasted on treating a condition that no longer existed.

During case discovery, questions were raised about the stuttering nature of Ms. Nell's decompensation. Why had her oxygenation improved before finally crashing? This pattern was entirely compatible with fat embolism. The first and milder manifestation was caused by a smaller embolism that had obstructed peripheral vessels in the lungs before a larger piece of fat occluded the main pulmonary artery shutting off any chance of survival. Had her doctors at the surgical center moved quickly and transferred her to a large referral hospital, she might have survived. Treating presumed asthma and waiting to transfer her to a small local hospital were mistakes that had a fatal consequence.

Also, several questions arose about the center's ability to address an emergency. To receive state licensure, it had the prerequisite staff training and equipment, but before Ms. Nell's disaster, none of the doctors or nurses on duty that day had ever participated in a resuscitation at the center. A few patients might have had transiently low blood pressure, but they usually responded to extra fluid. CPR was a totally different matter. Since the center was an island, in effect, there was no chance of soliciting help from more experienced hospital staff.

COMMENTARY

Over the past two decades, we have seen an exponential growth in the number of independent procedure and surgery centers in the US. Well over half of diagnostic and surgical procedures of all kinds are now performed outside the hospital setting. At first glance, it would seem to be a reasonable development. Surgical centers offer convenience and availability to patients who have been put off by the complexity of the urban medical center. Convenient parking, clean waiting rooms, eager staff, and easy scheduling are enticing. And most operators, unlike Dr. Bank, are highly experienced, since they carry out the same procedures at the same place every day. For the vast majority of low-risk patients, surgeries and colonoscopies and the like can be carried out safely in such an environment.

The reason for the proliferation of surgical centers is, like most things in modern medicine, a matter of money. Reimbursement for procedures is made in two parts, the technical and the professional components. The former is payment for the infrastructure including supplies, drugs, facilities and staff who participate in the procedure or operation. This is usually the far larger portion of the payment and in the past was provided to the hospitals where the procedures or operations occurred. The professional component is the fee paid to the operating physician, with a separate payment to the anesthesiologist. These fees are more tightly controlled and far smaller than the technical fee.

As the number of procedures increased and professional fees shrank, it didn't take long for doctors to figure out that they could make more money if they took their work out of the hospital and into the facilities they owned. There they could control costs, run an efficient schedule, and optimize income by reducing overhead compared to the bloated and over-administered hospital. When these enterprises proved to be cash cows, the rush was on. Quickly hospitals were deserted by just about every surgeon who didn't need Big Medicine to practice their trade. Joint replacements, cataract surgery, colonoscopies, and plastic surgery are just a few examples of the high revenue procedures that have moved out of hospitals.

To the unwitting patient public, all of this seemed like an excellent idea, and as stated above, for the most part it was. However, there are a few questions. First, what is the quality of the facilities? Although there is oversight by state licensing agencies, there is generally less supervision at these procedure mills than at hospitals. As we saw with Dr. Bank, physicians without the greatest skills, including those who have been censured, may find a home in sketchy centers.

By operating outside the hospital, the services offered at satellite centers don't necessarily have high clinical value. In fact, many offer services like stem cell injections, or laser back surgery, which have little or no proven value and would not pass muster at a hospital with circumspect physician governance.

Patient selection is also problematic. Which criteria determine whether a patient is or is not a suitable candidate for a procedure at a facility outside the hospital? The truth is that none of our professional organizations have addressed this question, and so the answer is left to the doctors, who are highly motivated to perform the profitable procedure.

Some of the cases where harm has been discovered are truly egregious. Consider the case of a 60-year-old woman with hypertension, diabetes, sleep apnea, COPD and obesity who suffered a respiratory arrest after having laser back surgery at an ambulatory center in a strip mall. The physician who "cleared" her for the procedure made no recommendation about where the surgery should be performed. If he had insisted on a hospital setting, this patient would not have had the operation at all. Worthless laser back surgery was not a sanctioned procedure at any hospital in her area.

And the most compelling concern is that a prompt response to an emergency is simply not possible in surgical centers. They are not equipped or staffed to effectively treat a severe complication. They may tout transfer to a hospital as their bailout, but it is a hollow solution. In most dire medical emergencies, time is of the essence. Getting the patient to a facility that can deal with the complication within an hour is a feat, and even that is usually inadequate. And as we saw in Ms. Nell's case, the hospital chosen as the haven was itself unable to deal with her heart-lung emergency, and a second transfer was totally unfeasible.

CONCLUSION

Like nearly every other adult in the US, I have had a procedure in an outpatient facility. I was not particularly enthusiastic about the idea, given the concerns illustrated in this story, but I had no choice. My insurance company wouldn't pay for the procedure to be done at a hospital because it was much more expensive. Since I wanted my own doctor to do the work, I had to take the outpatient option. And the truth is that I did fine and was entirely satisfied with the overall experience. I had a great surgical result and no complications. Same story for my wife, other family members, and many of my patients. However, most of the people reading this account don't have the luxury of being able to do research to understand how much risk they are incurring by having their procedure at the Podunk Ambulatory Center, particularly if they have medical problems that might be exacerbated by the stress of surgery and anesthesia.

PATIENT ADVICE

The moral of this story for potential patients is clear: choosing the place to have your care in non-emergent situations is serious business. The essential points to consider are your general and cardiovascular health, the reputation and expertise of the operator, the benefits and the risks of the procedure, and the center's facilities and staffing, especially its ability to respond to an emergency in-house and with urgent transfer.

As professional fees continue to be slashed, physician groups will be ever more motivated to capture the technical component of common procedures. Therefore, this is another situation in which a thorough conversation with your trusted healthcare provider can be enormously helpful in selecting not only the best consultants but also the best care venues to maximize your chances of a good outcome. Good decisions will help you avoid another potential pitfall while navigating a healthcare system that cares more about profits than about you.

Story 12: Physician Reimbursement and Perverse Incentives

"Do as much as possible for the patient and as little as possible to the patient." —Bernard Lown, MD

NARRATIVE

Mr. East was a 60-year-old Caucasian man described by his family as a workaholic. He was an accountant who owned his firm and ran it like a drill sergeant. He demanded hard work and perfection from everyone who worked for him, and that probably explains why he turned employees over faster than the hamburger chef at Wendy's. Aside from his aggressive personality, Mr. East had few risk factors for cardiac disease. He exercised, though not regularly, and didn't eat particularly well despite his wife's admonitions. But he had no family history of coronary artery disease. His parents had lived well into their nineties and died of "old age." Seeing a cardiologist was considered unnecessary by his internist, but Mr. East insisted, perpetually obsessed as he was with the possibility of dropping dead suddenly as a couple of his friends recently had, one on a tennis court next to where Mr. East himself had been playing doubles. After that trauma, he decided on his own to make an appointment with Dr. Silver, a local cardiologist listed as a "Top Doc" in a city magazine.

Mr. East's personality included time urgency; he just couldn't stand wasting time on anything, even a doctor's appointment he had chosen to make on his own. Which is why he was angry when the secretary at Dr. Silver's office told him that the doctor was detained in the catheterization laboratory. She couldn't tell Mr. East how long he would have to wait, but she hoped it wouldn't be much longer.

Over the next hour, Mr. East became impatient until he worked himself into a frenzy. He stormed up to the reception desk and announced he was leaving. Just then, Dr. Silver appeared, wearing a wrinkled scrub suit, a surgical cap, and a face mask down around his throat. Dr. Silver apologized profusely and asked his nurse to prepare Mr. East so he could be seen "promptly." The nurse escorted Mr. East into an examination room, took his vital signs, reviewed his medication and problem list, and performed an electrocardiogram. She departed, assuring Mr. East that Dr. Silver would be in "soon."

Apparently "promptly" and "soon" meant something different to Dr. Silver and his nurse because Mr. East sat on the examination table for another thirty minutes before Dr. Silver arrived. He placed his stethoscope on Mr. East's chest and briefly checked his pulses before turning to the computer.

Over his shoulder, Dr. Silver told Mr. East that everything looked to be in good order, and that his current situation was stable. He then paused, apparently having discovered something interesting in the medical record. He saw that Mr. East had gone to a free-standing testing center to get a calcium score. This score is determined using a scan in which the amount of calcium in and around the coronary arteries can be quantified. It is used as a predictor of coronary artery blockages and, when positive, suggests the need for further testing.

When Dr. Silver asked about the reason for the test, Mr. East said he had read about it on the internet and several of his friends had had one. He asked his primary care doctor to order it for him. He had been surprised that his insurance company refused to pay for it, but he was concerned enough to pay the $400 bill out of pocket. After the test, his primary care doctor told him that he had some calcium in his heart but that it was a normal aging thing, and he had forgotten about it.

Noticing Dr. Silver's look of concern, Mr. East began to pepper him with questions about the test results, what they meant and what should be done next. Dr. Silver was in a hurry. He was almost two full hours behind in his outpatient schedule and a randomly high calcium score was going to take a lot of explaining to a worried patient. Instead of addressing Mr. East's concerns in detail, Dr. Silver hurried his replies and concluded by telling Mr. East that if he was really worried about the possibility of coronary artery disease, his best choice would be to have more cardiac testing including a stress test with nuclear imaging, an echocardiogram and a heart rhythm monitor. When Mr. East asked questions about those tests, Dr. Silver again flew through the details. He told Mr. East that the secretary at the desk would give him a brochure that would include frequently asked questions, pictures and diagrams. She would also help him find a date and time for the tests. It would likely take about a month to have them all completed.

Dr. Silver logged off the computer, went to the door, and placed his hand on the doorknob, even as Mr. East continued to ask questions. After a few more monosyllabic answers, Dr. Silver left the room. Mr. East dressed and left the examination room feeling deeply dissatisfied with Dr. Silver's care, his demeanor, and his recommendations.

Mr. East was not about to let the issue drop or to proceed with a battery of tests he knew little about. He needed answers and if Dr. Silver wouldn't supply them, he would move on to another doctor. A recent commercial he had seen during the evening news pointed out that his local community hospital had recently opened a new catheterization laboratory, and they had recruited some expert doctors to join their staff, including a few who were "Top Docs" just like Dr. Silver.

It took only a few days to arrange an appointment with one of the interventional cardiologists, a young woman named Dr. Wynn. On arrival, Mr. East was promptly taken to an examination room. Within five minutes, Dr. Wynn appeared, dressed nicely in a clean white coat, with a stethoscope around her neck. When she asked how Mr. East had found his way to her office, he explained that he was unhappy with his previous cardiologist. He needed to talk about his heart problems and ask questions so he could make an informed decision.

Dr. Wynn's demeanor, like her dress, was distinctly different from Dr. Silver's. She spent time with Mr. East, examining him carefully, reviewing all his records, and then sitting down and explaining to him what the calcium score meant and what could be done about it. Calcium in a coronary artery meant there was plaque, but the test couldn't quantify how diseased the vessel might be. She told Mr. East that a cardiac catheterization was his best choice. It would provide definitive information, and if he had a blockage in any of his arteries, she would be able to open it up with a balloon and a stent. She explained the procedure to Mr. East in detail, answering his many questions. At the end, she told him she could schedule the test at her hospital at a convenient time and without more than a few days' wait.

Mr. East was encouraged by his interaction with this new cardiologist. Granted, he knew little about her, but judging by her demeanor and clear explanations, he was confident she would do a good job. He scheduled the catheterization before he left the office.

As promised, the procedure was well arranged and organized. He had his pre-procedure lab work and was able to register at intake quickly. During the procedure itself, he was well sedated and had minimal discomfort. Dr. Wynn was able to place a catheter into his wrist, thread it into his heart and inject dye to visualize his coronary arteries. Two of the three major coronary arteries were disease-free, but she identified a "significant" blockage in the right coronary artery. As discussed, and stipulated in the consent form he had signed, she expertly dilated the vessel and placed a stent. Mr. East was able to go home that very evening on a few new medications, feeling like a new man.

CASE EXPLANATION

This story may seem to have arrived at a successful conclusion, but the medical care system failed Mr. East several times, and in each case, it was because of perverse incentives.

Let's start at the beginning. Mr. East was one of millions of people we refer to as the "worried well," usually advantaged people who spend a good deal of their time obsessing about their health. Mr. East didn't have a cardiac problem, but because of aggressive advertising and peer pressure, he became afraid that he had coronary artery disease and was susceptible to sudden death. That prompted him to pester his primary care doctor to order a scan that would tell him if he had calcium in his coronary arteries and how much. Several of his friends had had the test and that convinced Mr. East that it was right for him.

The test was completely unnecessary. Mr. East had a normal cholesterol level, didn't smoke or have diabetes, and had no family history of coronary artery disease. The test was made available because it was a money-maker for the hospital, which could collect the entire fee directly from the patient without having to deal with a health insurance company that would discount the payment as it did with all tests. In this case, the insurance company simply refused to pay any portion of the fees for performing the test or interpreting it.

The primary care doctor shared the report with Mr. East and, given his good general health and lack of symptoms, minimized the results. That didn't sit well with Mr. East, who found his way to Dr. Silver, a doctor in a hurry, who failed to explain the test findings and provide reassurance. Instead, he suggested a battery of needless follow-up tests that he knew would be normal but would generate practice revenue. Seeing and testing healthy patients is a good way to keep your work units up without breaking a sweat.

Dr. Silver's behavior in the office put Mr. East off to the point of looking for another cardiologist. Why was Dr. Silver so abrupt? It so happened that Dr. Silver, as he did so often, overbooked himself in the catheterization laboratory that morning. When the procedures took longer than expected, he was terribly late to start his office hours and faced a waiting room full of anxious patients and a perturbed staff. He had to hurry through each appointment. When he saw Mr. East and established that he had a normal examination and electrocardiogram, he was surprised by the calcium test result. Dr. Silver sensed that Mr. East was an anxious soul, and that he was going to be inundated with questions. He did his best to answer a few and then fled the examination room while instructing Mr. East to read a brochure and schedule more tests.

Predictably, Mr. East sought care elsewhere. He stumbled onto an opportunistic interventional cardiologist who was smart enough to understand that he needed to be stroked and reassured before he would consent to a catheterization. She was right, and the test went forward without incident, including a revascularization using a stent placed in the middle portion of the right coronary artery. Mr. East transferred his care to his new cardiologist and hopefully lived happily ever after. But let's more carefully examine the path that brought Mr. East to the catheterization laboratory.

Mr. East was a worried patient who happened to be relatively affluent and therefore had access to whatever medical care he desired. Because of his constant state of anxiety about his heart, Mr. East decided to have an unnecessary calcium test. He persuaded his primary care doctor to order a scan that yielded a moderately high value. As mentioned, this test implies but does not prove the presence of coronary artery blockages. If the calcium score is high, it may mandate another test, like a stress test or a catheterization to see if the vessels are critically diseased. Because it is not a decisive study, medical insurance companies won't pay for it. Why should they when they know that a positive result will mean they have to pay for a definitive study like a stress test or a catheterization? Why not just cut to the chase and put the patient on a treadmill if it's clinically indicated?

Instead of reassuring Mr. East that he only needed to exercise, keep his cholesterol and blood pressure under control and refrain from smoking, Dr. Silver fanned the flames by telling Mr. East that he needed more cardiac tests. He then hurried out of the examination room, failing to provide Mr. East with enough information to help him decide whether to have the tests and what the results might mean. Dr. Silver was in a rush because he had been late for office hours. He wanted to do as many procedures as he could squeeze into his schedule to maximize his work units and thus his salary and bonus.

In the absence of symptoms or significant risk factors for coronary artery disease, there was no reason to order more tests. With a low pre-test probability of disease, the likelihood of a false positive test is almost as high as that of a true positive. Dr. Silver was simply turning the crank for his practice. He was savvy enough to know how to code the tests so that Mr. East's medical insurance company would approve a payment that was many times greater than the actual cost of the studies. A win for the practice's coffers.

Mr. East's next cardiologist, Dr. Wynn, was even more guileful. She didn't give Mr. East the option to have non-invasive tests but instead recommended a cardiac catheterization. Her motivation to do so was also perverse. Her hospital had hired her on the premise that she would bring her patients to the newly built, high-overhead catheterization laboratory. The window to prove herself and satisfy her overlords was short and Mr. East was a perfect prospect for her purposes. He was generally healthy and had excellent cardiac function, and his catheterization would be low risk. Dr. Wynn didn't expect to find much coronary artery disease, but the $10,000 test would only take a half hour or so. The administrators would not only be proud of her, but more cases would bolster her argument for a higher salary.

But Dr. Wynn's luck got even better. Mr. East had a right coronary artery lesion. If she stood on her head when she looked at the images and used her imagination, she could convince herself that the vessel was more than 70 percent occluded with diminished flow. Vessels stenosed by that much or more are assumed to be at risk for complete occlusion and so Dr. Wynn could justify placing a stent that doubled the cost of the procedure. Not only was the procedure successful, but Mr. East was ecstatic about the outcome. He felt he had been right all along in pursuing an invasive study. He was a new man. Mr. East would become an indentured patient in Dr. Wynn's practice and he would sing her praises to his wealthy friends and clients who could consult Dr. Wynn. And why not refer people to her? She had saved his life by sticking catheters into his heart and then jamming a stent into a coronary artery that never should have been touched. It was only by the grace of God that the artery didn't shut down and cause a heart attack or death.

COMMENTARY

This story, one that I came upon during a second opinion consultation, is not only about Mr. East's flawed management. It's also meant to illustrate how healthcare providers are paid for what they do, and how this negatively influences patient care.

As our modern profession emerged decades ago, the payment model was simple. You went to the doctor, he or she performed a service for which you paid a fee, usually in cash, but perhaps in kind with a chicken or a pie. It was not uncommon for doctors to provide "professional courtesy" and forgive the cost of care for other healthcare providers or their families or for people in real need. You might be surprised to learn that professional courtesy is no longer permissible. We are obliged to bill all patients under penalty of losing our credentials. And doctors who want to volunteer at clinics frequently can't do so because there is no way to pay for their malpractice insurance, unfortunately a necessary precaution even when treating patients for free.

As the cost of medicine increased, direct fee-for-service payment was no longer feasible. Although you might have been asked to pay the doctor a portion of the bill (a co-payment), you were expected to have some form of insurance to defray the bulk of the cost. These insurance policies were usually available as an employment benefit that was not a burden to employers when prices were modest. That system functioned well for several years, as long as practices remained small and simple, and the process for submitting bills to insurance companies and federal agencies like Medicare was straightforward.

Things started to change when every aspect of medical care became much more expensive and specialized, and it became clear that physicians could no longer supervise and administer their private practices. As the complexities multiplied, control had to be ceded to large practice groups, healthcare systems, or private equity firms. Practice acquisitions accelerated dramatically as regulation increased, placing physicians in greater jeopardy for noncompliance.

As doctors were disconnected from individual patient billing, the conundrum became how best to compensate physicians fairly. Despite multiple attempts, that problem has never been solved. The most obvious solution would be to continue to pay physicians a percentage of the revenue they generate, deducting the practice's overhead. The problem with this approach is that some physicians generate higher revenue not because they work harder, but because the things they do are paid at a higher rate than other tasks. Consider how much more money is paid to an interventional cardiologist who puts in expensive stents than to a general cardiologist who spends all day in the office, seeing patients for a low per-visit fee.

The next idea was to assign work units to various tasks so that each person in the practice would be able to benefit if they worked hard enough. Deciding which tasks are entitled to higher revenue is extremely complicated, especially since the cardiologists in the trenches get little or no credit for referring patients to their high-end colleagues. On the other hand, interventional cardiologists and electrophysiologists train longer than their general cardiology colleagues with the expectation of a higher salary.

Work unit allocation is further complicated when trying to incorporate non-patient-care activity into the equation. Many physicians have heavy administrative and teaching and research responsibilities, which generate little if any money for the practice or hospital but add prestige and reputation that benefits everyone. How much those activities are worth in work units for a compensation calculation has been hotly debated.

Most recently, nonphysician compensation "experts" have advocated for "value-based" compensation. In effect, doctors would be paid more if the care they rendered was of high quality. What is lacking is any idea of how to calculate care quality. Some groups have started by examining how often their practitioners refer patients to consultants, because referrals cost money, especially if the consultant recommends sophisticated tests or procedures. The irony is that stubborn refusal to refer frequently reflects ignorance of the importance of getting help before a case turns sour. Another touted idea is to restrict referral to "less expensive consultants," that is specialists who don't order as many tests. This strategy ignores the fact that some consultants need to order more tests because of the complexity of their referrals.

Gauging outcomes would of course be the key to any reimbursement paradigm but figuring out the most relevant outcomes and how any individual practitioner contributed to a good or bad outcome is difficult if not impossible. This is especially true in this era of fragmented care, in which whether a patient lives or dies can be the doings of one of a dozen caregivers. Furthermore, our patients, especially the elderly, don't have simple diseases. They have a multitude of co-morbidities, have numerous tests, and take several medications, all of which have a major impact on mortal or morbid outcomes.

At one point, the suggestion was made that patient satisfaction might be a good metric on which to base physician payment until it was shown in several studies that patients' opinions of their doctors have nothing to do with competence or quality. Holding a patient's hand is always reassuring to the patient, even if your treatment caused him to stop breathing.

After all is said and done, the system of payment that makes the most sense is a fixed salary based on training, job description, and seniority, with an opportunity for a modest, incentivizing bonus. It would consider the value the physician brings to the enterprise and compensate for time teaching and doing research, activities that are reputationally valuable. There would be regional differences because of the cost of living and other factors, but trainees would have a firm idea of what their compensation might be when they, as medical students, decide which specialty to pursue.

Implicit in this approach is doing away with the huge debt that new doctors bear by forgiving loans for those willing to practice for smaller salaries and/or in deprived areas. Choice of specialty would be less dependent on how much money could be made to repay the hundreds of thousands of dollars of debt our young doctors face.

Will this system work? It has been in place in other countries for decades and works well when the compensation packages have been well thought out and justified. But implementing it would mean that physicians would have to surrender the "get-rich" expectation so many have as they enter the workforce, as well as jeopardizing sufficient cash flow to pay back high interest student loans.

CONCLUSION

Compared to other people in our society, doctors make a lot of money. However, given the length of their training and their level of responsibility, they deserve to be paid well. The problem we are addressing in this story is that doctors, like other human beings, want to be compensated at a fair level, and they are not. Consider that a senior doctor, one who wrote the textbook in her sub-specialty, is paid $150 to see a new patient in the office, a task that takes at least ninety minutes. That is the same fee paid to a young rhythm specialist one day out of her training, and considerably less than what our plumber is paid to examine our home's water heater. And what about that senior orthopedic surgeon performing joint replacements for which he receives about $180 per hour, or roughly one-fifth of what a senior partner in a law firm bills hourly? These low Medicare prescribed rates have not kept pace with inflation, and have been further reduced in recent years, placing even more fiscal pressure on physicians and other healthcare professionals.

To compensate for inadequate fees, doctors do the expected thing, which is to ramp up the number of procedures they carry out to maintain their wage. Consider that as the compensation for a catheter ablation procedure to treat atrial fibrillation has fallen by 20 to 30 percent, the number of procedures carried out in the US has increased by a factor of 10. That isn't because the procedure is any more safe or effective than it was five years ago, or that there are so many more people doing ablations or patients who need them. It is simply a matter of guns and butter economics. The problem in medical care is that patients are being subjected to procedures they may not need or for which realistic alternatives are available if only doctors were compensated fairly for non-procedural care.

I suspect that as the current generation of senior doctors passes the torch to its successors, the contentiousness surrounding compensation models will diminish. Newly minted doctors won't know what it was like to be valued as professionals and to be paid fairly for their work. Instead, they will punch a time clock, work shifts, and receive a salary that will be considerably lower than that of a hospital administrator, but considerably higher than the median US income. How that will appeal to the patient public and to bright young people making career choices, and how well we can maintain even a modicum of quality care under such circumstances very much remains to be seen.

PATIENT ADVICE

It is not unreasonable to ask how much your doctor is being paid for the work she or he does. Admittedly, the answer is complicated. Various factors determine physician fees, but you will be surprised to learn how little of what is billed for procedures and office visits finds its way to the physician's paycheck. The hospital bill for a total hip procedure may be six figures, but after insurance company discounts and overhead payments, about 1 percent goes to the surgeon.

Unfortunately, some doctors take advantage of patients by carrying out unnecessary or marginally necessary procedures. The only way to steer clear of a procedure mill is once again to trust your physician who makes the referral to send you to the most competent and compassionate healthcare provider available and accessible under the terms of your healthcare insurance, supplemented by whatever you can discover about outcomes for that provider and the institution where they work. Paradoxically, it is often the consultant who recommends procedures only when absolutely necessary who is usually the busiest and the most technically proficient. The wise physician knows that doing less may be the best thing for the patient and for herself.

Story 13: The Medical Education Fiasco

"Today, somebody is going to be referred to the doctor who registered the lowest passing board score of all time." —Anonymous

NARRATIVE

Our story takes place about fifteen years ago. Mrs. Uler was a 48-year-old Caucasian woman who worked hard at home managing a large house and caring for three children, the oldest of whom was college-bound. She exercised when she could and kept to a reasonable diet. She was in good general health with no major medical issues but had a few annoying problems. As a girl, she had what her mother called "athlete's foot" and, over the years, despite using topical medication, she developed a fungal infection in her toenails. Besides making it hard to trim her nails, the problem made her feet unsightly, such that she never took her shoes off in public and never wore open-toe sandals. This was a particular problem in the summer when she and her family enjoyed trips to the shore, and she wanted to walk on the beach. She had come up with several workarounds, like wearing waterproof boat shoes so she could go into the surf, and picking sandals that covered the tips of her toes. Dr. Yeats, her primary care doctor, had suggested a highly effective oral medication. Mrs. Uler was reluctant to take a drug with potential side effects and drug interactions for what she perceived to be merely a cosmetic issue. She was particularly concerned because she had read that the drug could damage the liver, and her mother had died in hepatic failure, albeit with a history of alcohol abuse.

Her other nagging issue was seasonal allergies. Every spring, as soon as flowers began to bloom, she would start to sneeze. At times, her nasal congestion was intolerable and disturbed her sleep. She regularly had what she referred to as "allergy days" when she was almost completely nonfunctional. The only way to get any relief from the runny nose, sore throat and headache was to take Benadryl, at the time the most widely used antihistamine. Its major side-effect was sedation, so when Mrs. Uler had her worst allergy days, she had to resort to taking it, essentially knocking her out of commission, leaving her barely able to stay awake, let alone carry out her usual household and family chores. Being sedated was better than wiping her nose and sneezing all day.

While watching TV with her husband one evening, just as the allergy season was upon her, Mrs. Uler saw a commercial advertising the first nonsedating antihistamine, a prescription drug called Seldane. According to the happy people in the commercial, the drug was highly effective for suppressing allergy symptoms and was particularly useful for those who, like Mrs. Uler, had seasonal allergies. She wrote down the name of the drug and the next day called Dr. Yeats' office to inquire about the availability of this new product. The nurse with whom she spoke told Mrs. Uler that since it was a prescription drug, she would need to be seen in the office before starting it. However, she promised to pass the inquiry on to Dr. Yeats. Since she had an upcoming appointment, the nurse was sure that the doctor would talk to her about it then.

Dr. Yeats was a middle-aged woman who had immigrated to the US from Ireland with her family. Hers was an American success story. Through hard work and perseverance, she had managed to attend an Ivy League university and then a topflight medical school, where she earned not only an MD, but also a PhD in microbiology. She was certain that she would end up as an academic infectious disease specialist focusing on research, but during her general internal medicine residency, she realized that she liked the challenge of general practice and eventually took a job as an internist in a small practice.

The first few years were exciting for Dr. Yeats, but with time, she became overwhelmed by the clerical and administrative parts of her job. She found herself spending an inordinate amount of time maintaining the medical record and interacting with stubborn payers. Between all of that and her patient care, Dr. Yeats had no time to read or attend conferences, and though she had agreed to mentor medical students, she simply had little opportunity to teach the young doctors when they were in the office with her. It didn't matter because she didn't have much cutting-edge knowledge to share with them. She was ashamed to admit that most of the new information she gathered came from snippets on the internet or news headlines and not from major medical journals that accumulated in piles in her home office.

The drug detailers were another pitifully poor source of information for Dr. Yeats. Pharmaceutical companies hired attractive young people to visit doctors' offices and hospitals to make physicians aware of newly approved and marketed drugs. They typically asked for about ten minutes to sit with the physician, to briefly explain the new medication, and answer questions. The goal was to encourage the doctor to try the medication on a few patients and hope that the results were good enough to make her an adopter. To move the process along, samples were provided to the office to help get patients started for no charge, a further enticement. These days most hospitals and practices limit drug representatives' access to their physicians on the presumption that it induces inappropriate use of new and expensive drugs, but samples are still expected and welcome.

By coincidence, the drug company representative who was promoting terfenadine, trade name Seldane, visited Dr. Yeats a few days before Mrs. Uler's appointment. She came with a couple of journal articles and a nicely produced brochure that summarized the results of the pivotal trials that were carried out to support the FDA approval of Seldane, in which it had outperformed Benadryl in stopping runny noses and itchy eyes, and most importantly, didn't cause sedation. She explained the dosing recommendations and, by regulation, pointed out the drug's major adverse effects and its potential for interactions with other drugs, while emphasizing Seldane's lack of a sedative effect. Dr. Yeats was impressed with the efficacy and safety results, in particular Seldane's good tolerance, and promised the salesperson that she would consider using the drug in some of her patients. The samples would be particularly helpful.

When Mrs. Uler came for her visit, she complained about her allergies and her frustrations with Benadryl and wanted to know what Dr. Yeats thought about the Seldane idea. Dr. Yeats told her that she had received Mrs. Uler's message and agreed that it was worth a try. She instructed Mrs. Uler about dosing and potential side effects and gave her enough samples for a month, reminding Mrs. Uler that the drug was more expensive than Benadryl, which would be an issue if she decided to use it long-term.

Mrs. Uler had an excellent experience with the Seldane samples. She experienced no side effects, and her allergy symptoms were vastly improved. Best of all, she could take it once or twice a day to prevent an allergy attack without feeling at all sleepy.

When Mrs. Uler returned to see Dr. Yeats, she was grateful and upbeat, so much so that she told Dr. Yeats she had decided to do something about the fungus infection in her toenails. Dr. Yeats happily provided her with a prescription for a generic and widely available anti-fungal drug called ketoconazole that worked wonders for previous patients. The best part was that Mrs. Uler would have to use the drug for only ten days to get a good therapeutic result.

Once again, Mrs. Uler had a good drug response. She watched as new, clear nail grew from the cuticle, pushing out the diseased portion to where she would soon be able to clip the ugly fungus completely away. All was going well until one late afternoon about seven days later when she started having intense dizzy spells that made her feel as if she were going to pass out. She waited until her husband returned from work to ask his advice. Fortunately, he didn't hesitate to whisk her off to the local emergency room.

Mrs. Uler lost consciousness in a wheelchair as she was brought into the ER. She was carried onto a bed and attended to by two doctors and a host of nurses and other staff. They placed her on a cardiac monitor and thereupon observed some of the most abnormal heart rhythms any of them had ever seen. Their first thought was that the reading was a movement artifact, but they quickly concluded that it was real, and it was very serious.

During the long runs of the arrhythmia, Mrs. Uler had no recordable blood pressure so the staff started CPR and placed stat pages to the anesthesia and cardiology departments. Fortunately, one of the cardiac rhythm specialists was doing late rounds in the hospital and ran down to the ER. As soon as he saw the monitor strips, he asked for magnesium and lidocaine, which were administered intravenously. Before the anesthesiologist needed to intubate Mrs. Uler, the abnormal heart rhythms stopped, her blood pressure rapidly recovered, and she started to wake up.

The ER doctors and staff were finally able to take a deep breath and sort out what had happened. According to the cardiologist, Mrs. Uler's cardiac arrhythmia arose from the bottom chambers of her heart, the ventricles, and it was called Torsade de Pointes. The arrhythmia occurred in association with an abnormality of the heart's electrical system commonly caused by medication or an electrolyte abnormality. The latter was ruled out with routine blood tests, so the focus turned to Mrs. Uler's drug history. They learned from Mr. Uler that his wife was taking two medications, Seldane and ketoconazole. A quick computer search uncovered the problem.

Ketoconazole inhibits an enzyme that metabolizes terfenadine so that concentrations of the drug increase several-fold. At very high concentrations, Seldane interferes with the cardiac electrical system and causes the exact arrhythmia Mrs. Uler had manifest. The two drugs that the cardiologist had ordered and administered in the ER were the correct antidotes and explained the rapid cessation of the arrhythmia. Mrs. Uler was admitted to the hospital to keep a close watch on her heart rhythm until the Seldane was completely out of her system.

Mrs. Uler's recovery was complete and by the next morning, she was sitting up in bed having breakfast when she was visited by Dr. Yeats. She had gotten a message that Mrs. Uler had been admitted through the ER and had suffered a life-threatening arrhythmia. Dr. Yeats had gone through her chart to discover her error and had come to see Mrs. Uler to apologize for the mistake. Seldane was a relatively new drug and she had not taken the time to learn about its drug interactions before she subsequently prescribed ketoconazole. Dr. Yeats was relieved beyond measure that Mrs. Uler would recover without permanent harm. She hoped that Mrs. Uler would allow Dr. Yeats to continue to care for her, but reassured Mr. and Mrs. Uler that she would understand if she went elsewhere.

Mrs. Uler ultimately chose to stop taking Seldane and ketoconazole and live with her fungus toenails. She also chose to continue her care with Dr. Yeats, having forgiven her for the prescribing error and its near catastrophic consequences. With no treatment, her allergies roared back. She was afraid of taking Seldane again, even without ketoconazole. She resumed Benadryl but was even more unhappy about sleepiness. Fortunately, it was only weeks later that the successor to Seldane, Allegra, came on the market. It was thoroughly tested for cardiac safety, and it was also found to be as effective as its predecessor. Dr. Yeats had learned her lesson and before prescribing it, read everything she could find about the new drug. She was reassured that it was cardiac-safe, and with confidence offered it to Ms. Uler and other patients who were happy with the good results and lack of side effects.

CASE EXPLANATION

What happened to Mrs. Uler was a direct result of the inadequacy of continuing medical education. Dr. Yeats was a bright, well-intentioned physician who chose a medical specialty, general internal medicine, that eats doctors for lunch. Primary care medicine is, by its nature, impossible to practice well. Family physicians are pressured to see dozens of patients every day, leaving almost no time for their continuing education. Medical science advances apace, and good doctors like Dr. Yeats simply can't keep up. They have little time to read the literature or attend conferences or grand rounds, and yet they are expected to possess knowledge in several medical specialties in which advances occur at warp speed. As we saw in the story about physician burnout, anxiety and depression run very high in generalists who struggle to do the right thing.

In the present case, Dr. Yeats had the opportunity to prescribe a new drug for allergy symptoms. She was given articles from the medical literature by the drug representative. Never mind that those articles were skewed in favor of Seldane, because Dr. Yeats didn't have time to read them anyway before she gave samples to Mrs. Uler. Her "education" about Seldane came from a glance at a brochure and a few graphs, and information about how to dose the drug from a drug representative with a bachelor's degree in history.

Even worse, after the release of Seldane, and before Dr. Yeats prescribed it, the potentially fatal drug interaction with ketoconazole had been described and a few unexpected sudden cardiac deaths in relatively young people had been reported. Those deaths had prompted a "Dear Doctor" letter from the FDA warning physicians not to use the two drugs together. That letter had come across Dr. Yeats's desk twice in the months before the Uler debacle. When she was told about them later, she couldn't remember if she had even opened the envelope. She received so many messages that it was impossible to read most of them. In any case, that highly directed and important educational message had been ignored, and not only by Dr. Yeats. Data collected subsequently showed that the concomitant use of Seldane and ketoconazole actually increased after the warning letters had gone out to physicians. In other words, the most direct attempts to educate doctors, sending warning letters, failed miserably.

Before Mrs. Uler's calamity, Dr. Yeats was thinking about her long-term future as an internist. She was progressively dissatisfied with her routine, her long work hours, and even more by the lack of intellectual stimulation. She had no time to educate herself or others, or to delve into interesting cases, which she simply passed on to subspecialty consultants. She longed for the time she had spent in the research laboratory thinking about experiments and then executing them in a controlled environment. She missed the thrill of discovery and the pride she had felt when her work was selected for presentation at a prominent medical conference or for publication in a first-rate journal. Her experience with Mrs. Uler solidified her decision to leave her patients and seek employment in industry, where her research interests could be properly nurtured.

Dr. Yeats' greatest fear was that Mrs. Uler would bring a lawsuit against her for malpractice. That was the reason for her hospital visit and apology. She was relieved when Mrs. Uler resumed care with her office. A few months later, Dr. Yeats sent a form letter to Mrs. Uler and all of her patients announcing the closing of her clinical practice and her intention to pursue a career in industry. Mrs. Uler called Dr. Yeats to tell her she was grateful for the care she had received, and to offer best wishes for Dr. Yeats as she headed back into research medicine.

COMMENTARY

Medical education is in crisis. From the time very bright college graduates enter medical school to the end of their careers, learning is inconsistent and inadequate. The medical school curriculum has been tinkered with for years without a satisfactory result. Part of the problem is that most of the people who sit on curriculum committees have never been in a real practice situation. Thus, they are ignorant of the things that practicing doctors need to know.

Examples of this disconnect abound but consider that most medical schools teach nothing about business. Understanding billing, insurance, and budgets is integral to what a doctor needs to know to survive in clinical practice. It has been physician naivete in this regard that has led to their willingness to cede control of the financial end of their practices to administrators who know nothing about the core business of medicine.

Another disconnect is that doctors aren't taught how to use biostatistics to assess clinical research. Understanding the basic principles of how to interpret clinical trials is essential for physicians to help them evaluate the worth of new therapies or diagnostic methods as they are published in medical journals. How else can they decide which of hundreds of innovations to incorporate into their clinical practice? Without an understanding of how data are processed or analyzed, they can be influenced by bad science.

Medical writing is also glossed over and yet the ability to write a cogent letter about a patient or to communicate intelligently is essential to good patient care. If a doctor sends an unintelligible letter, she or he is presumed to be incompetent no matter how well they practice their craft. Instead of learning how to present patients coherently to their colleagues, and to write decipherable notes, medical students spend time learning a good deal of basic science that they will never use and soon forget. I spend a considerable amount of time correcting the grammar of trainees from prestigious medical schools who have completed research projects and written reports, hoping to have them published.

Though they will be overwhelmed with questions about diet from patients, medical students learn virtually nothing about nutrition. Literature abounds with information about the importance of certain nutrients to maintain good health that is virtually ignored in didactic lectures and on the wards. Instead, students and residents are subjected to endless social science seminars in which instructors struggle to convey to them what it takes to have a human interaction with a patient.

The quality of the educational settings is also of concern. When it finally dawned on leaders in medical education that we are doomed to have an insufficient number of doctors to care for our citizens, the response was to increase class sizes and open new medical schools. Increasing the size of a lecture hall or recruiting good teachers for the basic sciences was difficult, but finding high quality facilities for clinical teaching was even more daunting. What has emerged is a patchwork of second-rate community hospitals being proffered as "teaching facilities," in which medical students learn little from the harried doctors who work there. Some programs resort to using virtual reality training to substitute for direct patient contact. The diminished fund of knowledge and clinical experience for these disadvantaged students creates a learning deficit unlikely to be remedied as they progress in their medical training.

Internship and residency training is no better. Newly minted physicians rotate on a variety of acute care floors with an uneven degree of supervision and spotty teaching from faculty who are themselves expected to carry a heavy clinical load. Most of what they learn is from senior residents with little experience of their own. The emphasis is on learning how to do procedures, with very little time given over to teaching how to take a comprehensive history or perform a thorough physical examination. Looking at a blood smear or a urine sample in a microscope, formerly an intern's responsibility, has been jettisoned entirely.

After all the publicity about long work hours, and despite no evidence that working fewer hours improves patient outcomes, residents now work in shifts. This means they will never have the experience of being responsible for the complete care of a sick patient. They hand patients over to their colleagues no matter the situation. Handoffs themselves are problematic since students are not taught how to make a succinct and well-prepared patient presentation. They are not expected to be responsible for mistakes, and if an attending physician has the temerity to discipline a student or resident, there will certainly be repercussions.

Even though most trainees will spend a significant portion of their career in the office seeing patients, only a small percentage of their training occurs in the outpatient area, usually in an unsupervised charity clinic where they have no opportunity to deliver continuing or meaningful care or to have their mistakes corrected and their bedside behavior honed.

Knowledge of the literature is not expected of residents. Google or UpToDate provide facts quickly for specific patient problems, and residents almost never have the opportunity to delve deeply into the established literature. However, if they wish to apply for a fellowship in a sub-specialty, they are encouraged to perform some "research," which for them usually consists of producing case reports, small retrospective studies, or meta-analyses that waste time and journal pages. The "literature" now includes hundreds of barely credible "open access" journals that are happy to take your money to publish what amounts to worthless research results. Sifting through such material to find articles of worth adds to the difficulty of understanding the state of the art of any clinical problem and makes "keeping up with the literature" impossible.

Like their patients and hospital employees, interns and residents have suffered terribly during the epidemic of hospital closures, with sharp declines in patient volume before bankruptcy is finally declared. Consider the story of a struggling 125-bed suburban hospital that had an average census of eight patients serviced by eighteen primary care residents in the months before it closed for good, and the trainees cast adrift.

There is nothing much different in advanced clinical training or subspecialty fellowships. The saving grace here is that the skills and knowledge imparted are more focused and more likely to be used upon the completion of training. The problem is the emphasis on learning procedures that can generate revenue. Being able to do procedures and operations is what makes training graduates attractive job candidates, and that is how they will make enough money to repay loans and have a reasonable family life.

Cardiology fellows who are interested in my sub-specialty, cardiac arrhythmia treatment, spend hours upon hours in the cardiac ablation laboratory being schooled on how to move catheters in the body to deliver energy to ablate arrhythmia foci. They spend precious little time learning the nuts and bolts of actual electrophysiology practice. They learn next to nothing about antiarrhythmic drugs and how to prescribe them, even though almost every patient with a common arrhythmia needs drug treatment at some point in their care. Basic skills, like reading an electrocardiogram, the most common clinical test in cardiology, are poorly taught, if at all. The result is mistakes in interpretation that can have disastrous clinical consequences.

Perhaps the most egregious education gap is for doctors in practice. Primary care physicians, including internists like Dr. Yeats, are particularly disadvantaged for the reasons already discussed. The problem begins during their training, where time management is never taught. That deficit is magnified when they are drowned with clinical work, as all clinicians are. No one who is already working fourteen hours a day is going to attend conferences and when they do make it to Grand Rounds, they are likely to have to sit through an overly detailed explanation of a rare disease they have never seen and likely never will, all because the syndrome may be considered "interesting" by the meeting organizers.

Keeping up with the medical literature, now consisting of literally thousands of medical journals, is a torment, especially if the physician has not been provided with the rudimentary knowledge of how best to interpret the studies that might pertain to their patients. Nevertheless, they are expected to know "the guidelines" for the treatment of a hundred different diseases, directives put out by professional organizations that unwittingly expose doctors to lawsuits and censure whenever their care doesn't meet a standard not necessarily established by the best medical science.

Consider Dr. Yeats. Though she cared for hundreds of patients with allergic conditions, she was unaware of a new drug that had the potential to revolutionize their management. A drug representative and a patient who saw a television commercial gave her an introduction that was not only inadequate but downright dangerous.

At the same time that doctors struggle with accessing new information, they are also expected to study and take examinations on a regular basis to maintain their certification. Whether making doctors go through these exercises improves patient outcomes has never been established. In some cases, the burden of recertification can be enormous. Consider the case of the cardiac electrophysiologist who saved Mrs. Uler's life. He had achieved board certification in internal medicine, cardiovascular medicine and cardiac electrophysiology. If he chose to maintain his certification in all three, he would be required to study and take examinations for each of the three certifications every ten years on his own time and on his own dime.

CONCLUSION
"The young physician starts life with 20 drugs for each disease, and the old physician ends life with one drug for 20 diseases." —Sir William Osler

The ideal goal of the medical education process is to turn young, eager and well-intentioned young students into experienced, wise senior doctors with a large fund of knowledge and a real interest in making patients fare better. For whatever reason, we have lost our way—witnessed by the large number of doctors who are poorly informed, frustrated, and burned out.

We are left with the question of how to make this broken educational system work better. One might be tempted to simply throw up one's hands and say we are doomed. I don't agree. We can find a way to take young and correctly motivated people and give them the tools they need to be effective practitioners.

The medical school curriculum would be a good place to start. Curriculum committees need to enlist the help of practitioners in determining the best content and course instruction. This can't be a volunteer activity or part-time employment. Seasoned clinicians with research and teaching skills must be properly motivated to participate on a continuing basis.

Also needed is a much more realistic approach to graduate medical education, including residency and fellowship. Young doctors must be encouraged to learn not only about procedures and methods, but also how to continue to learn once they are in practice. We must emphasize the best things that doctors do, which is delivering compassionate care to patients, understanding the limitations of technology, and the importance of maintaining hope even when the disease is overwhelming. Mentorship is key, so improving the quality of what we loosely refer to as "teaching hospitals" is paramount. All of this will require an investment of capital and a thoughtful disbursement of those funds to places in the community where our young doctors are growing up.

PATIENT ADVICE

There are few things that patients can do to remedy the crisis of medical education. First, the public must clearly understand that the stakes here are high. Supporting legislators who understand the importance of subsidizing medical education at all levels is an important idea. We now know that well-endowed medical schools can suspend tuition, and more should be encouraged to do so. Unionization of house officers and attending physicians may bring education quality into better focus, for debate and improvement, and as such, deserves our backing.

Most importantly, we must be fully aware that if we don't change course and do a better job of educating people who are pursuing healthcare as a profession, not only will we have a shortage of providers, but those we have won't be equipped to take the best care of us.

Story 14: Acquisition Mania and the Private Equity Mess

"The role of private equity... is certainly to make money." —Thomas Stemberg

NARRATIVE

Mrs. Epps was a healthy and affluent 33-year-old woman who, with her husband, decided to buy a horse farm in a beautiful rural area. They moved there from a city condominium largely because they wanted to start a family and thought that having a country home, reasonably near excellent schools, would be a lifestyle advantage. Mr. Epps had ascended in his law firm to the point that he could work remotely at least three days a week, and his two-day commute was tolerable. Mrs. Epps was a potter who was looking forward to having her own art studio in their newly converted barn.

Mrs. Epps became pregnant shortly after their move. Her ob-gyn physician, a doctor she adored, was in residence at the University Hospital, but the couple was reassured that he would be able to see her as frequently as necessary at the university's satellite facility near their home. He also had privileges at the local community hospital and planned to be present at the delivery.

The pregnancy proceeded normally, and Mrs. Epps delivered her firstborn son without incident. Her university-based obstetrician was not in attendance, but a covering physician presided over the delivery and did an excellent job. The pediatrician in the labor room pronounced their new baby to be in good health.

The trouble started when, at the first well baby visit, their pediatrician heard a heart murmur. She referred the baby to a pediatric cardiologist, Dr. Herr, at the children's hospital in the city. Dr. Herr heard the same systolic murmur and immediately ordered an echocardiogram. The test confirmed that Baby Epps had congenital aortic stenosis, or a narrowing of the valve that opened to permit blood to leave the heart and travel to the general circulation. If the stenosis is severe, it can cause congestive heart failure, serious cardiac rhythm abnormalities, and in the worst cases, death.

Baby Epps's aortic stenosis was classified as only moderately severe; that is, the valve was not critically blocked. Dr. Herr outlined two options: fixing the valve through a catheter or replacing it with surgery. Given the baby's good health and age, he advised close clinical observation and medication to ease the pressure on the heart for the time being. He advised Mr. and Mrs. Epps of the symptoms and signs that would require a rapid response, that is speeding the baby to an emergency facility. Before buying their new farm, Mr. and Mrs. Epps had done their homework and knew exactly how long it would take them, or an ambulance, to get to the closest hospital, about six miles south of their home.

For the next several weeks, Baby Epps prospered. The family had frequent visits with Dr. Herr who was satisfied that the valve stenosis was not progressing and that the baby was reaching his growth and development milestones on time. The medications were keeping the load on the heart down to the point that the heart was functioning normally, and the walls were not thickening.

Dr. Herr told the parents that he was certain that a corrective procedure would be necessary at some point, but waiting and allowing the child to grow and develop would significantly lessen the risks of the valve replacement. The later they operated, the longer it would be until another operation was necessary to place a larger valve in the child's growing heart. Once again, he warned the parents about the possibility of heart failure and the need to respond quickly to any symptoms that might suggest a cardiac arrhythmia. He gave them his cell phone number and instructed them to call if they had any questions.

Mr. and Mrs. Epps's bedroom was only a few steps from the nursery, and they kept a baby monitor on their bedside table. They had become accustomed to hearing the baby cry in the middle of the night, hungry, wet, or both, and needing their ministration. So, on this stormy weekend night, Baby Epps's crying raised no alarm. Mr. Epps volunteered to take care of the baby's needs. He picked up Baby Epps in the dark and could tell immediately that his son was struggling to breathe. When he flicked on the overhead light, he was horrified to see that his son was blue, struggling in his arms. He called out for his wife who, after seeing the situation, ran back to their bedroom, found her cell phone, and called 911. She explained the situation to the operator and was reassured that help would arrive within minutes.

Though Mr. and Mrs. Epps had been told to respond to severe symptoms by summoning help, they had no idea how to make their baby better or resuscitate him. They simply paced the house, holding their distressed son, and listening for a siren. The response time ended up being only about five minutes. A paramedic and an EMT hurried through the front door, took the baby to a table in the foyer, and began to do CPR. They told the parents they would try to establish an airway and an IV and then take the baby to the nearest emergency room.

The crew called the emergency medicine service to report their situation and get medication orders and instructions. Unfortunately, neither of the responders had experience with pediatric intubation, so they had to settle for a face mask to deliver extra oxygen. Similarly, they were unable to insert an intravenous line and resorted to injecting medication into the baby's leg bone. Nothing they did seemed to help. Finally, they wrapped the baby in a heavy blanket and prepared to load him into the ambulance. They told the parents not to try to follow them, they would be moving very fast with emergency lights and siren. It would be best if they met them at the hospital ER as soon as they could get there.

Mr. and Mrs. Epps nodded their agreement and hurried into their bedroom to change. In only a few minutes, they had locked the house, gotten into their car, and taken off to the local hospital. Once in the hospital driveway, they followed signs to the ER and were shocked to find that it was closed. A sign on the shuttered door directed patients needing emergency assistance to a hospital fifteen miles away.

The couple jumped back into their car and located the alternate hospital on their GPS. While Mr. Epps drove like a man possessed, Mrs. Epps called the hospital and confirmed that their child had arrived. They realized that the ambulance crew had never intended to go to their local hospital; they knew that the ER there was closed and assumed Mr. and Mrs. Epps knew that as well and would travel to the next closest hospital.

Twenty nerve-wracking minutes later, Mr. and Mrs. Epps pulled into a parking space and sprinted into the ER. They were greeted by an older woman who reassured them that their child was being evaluated by the doctor who would be out to talk to them in a few minutes. After what seemed like hours, a young doctor came out to the waiting area. He asked several questions about the baby and then told Mr. and Mrs. Epps that he had managed to get a tube into the baby's lungs and inserted an IV and was giving him medication to help clear the fluid from his lungs. But Baby Epps was in severe heart failure and would need specialty care. Unfortunately, his hospital didn't have a pediatric department or a neonatal intensive care unit. The baby would need to get to the city children's hospital as soon as possible. With storms in the area, helicopter transport was not an option. The ambulance that had transported their son was still available. He suggested that the ambulance crew take their son to the city.

Mr. and Mrs. Epps were shocked. They had no idea of the dearth of medical care facilities in their area. They hadn't thought to intensively research the issue. They knew their excellent pediatrician was fully available to them for outpatient care and phone consultation, and they also knew there was a hospital with an emergency room minutes from their home. They never imagined being in dire straits with an infant son in extremis.

They asked the doctor to arrange for the transfer while Mr. Epps called Dr. Herr. He agreed with an immediate transfer to Children's Hospital and promised he would be there to take care of the baby when they arrived.

Baby Epps was breathing more easily and sleeping intermittently when they carried him out to the ambulance. The weather had gotten worse, but since it was late into the night, the ambulance crew reassured the parents that the trip would go quickly. To be extra safe, they had called in a veteran ambulance driver so the EMT and paramedic would be able to ride in the back with Baby Epps.

What the crew later related to Dr. Herr was that the first fifteen minutes of the trip had gone well. But suddenly, the baby's heart rhythm became erratic with multiple premature beats and runs of ventricular tachycardia that quickly deteriorated into a cardiac arrest. The crew began CPR and attempted to shock the heart back into a normal rhythm. They were successful at first, but within only a couple of minutes, the arrhythmias recurred. The cycle of arrhythmia and shock was repeated at least three of four times before the ambulance arrived at the children's hospital.

The resuscitation there, now supervised by Dr. Herr, went no better. Despite the use of multiple drugs and circulatory support, the baby's heart remained electrically unstable and eventually stopped completely. Mr. and Mrs. Epps arrived after the ER code had been called off and were greeted by Dr. Herr who explained that the delay in treating the heart failure had taken a terrible toll on Baby Epps's heart which had become irreversibly irritable and out of rhythm. Mr. and Mrs. Epps were inconsolable, unable to process the events of the worst night of their young lives.

CASE EXPLANATION

Baby Epps was diagnosed with congenital aortic stenosis. That means he was born with an abnormal heart valve that wouldn't open normally and allow blood to flow to his body. The pediatric resident who had examined the baby after his delivery didn't hear a murmur but by the nature of the lesion, it must have been audible if the doctor had been properly trained and listened carefully. The condition wasn't picked up until a more senior pediatrician heard the murmur and made a referral to a cardiology specialist. Appropriate testing confirmed the diagnosis, and because the stenosis was not critical, the cardiologist appropriately recommended conservative management until the baby was old enough to have a procedure to replace the valve.

Aortic stenosis is a treacherous disease because, despite best efforts, complications can occur without warning. The worst complication is death from an arrhythmia. But the sudden development of heart failure is another hazard. Baby Epps had both. For unclear reasons, the valve lesion acutely worsened, and blood could no longer be ejected from the ventricle. It backed up into Baby Epps's lungs, causing blood oxygenation to deteriorate. The heart, deprived of sufficient oxygen and under increased pressure, became electrically unstable. The arrhythmias worsened and finally resulted in a cardiac arrest.

Was Baby Epps's death avoidable? The doctors were correct in recommending conservative management. When waiting to replace a diseased heart valve, it is always a good idea to give the child a chance to grow and to defer the first of what could be several valve replacements over his or her life. After making that decision, physicians warned Mr. and Mrs. Epps to respond quickly to any sign or symptom of heart failure, which they did. What all of them failed to consider was the availability of emergency facilities in their neighborhood, a rural area, several miles from any large pediatric hospitals. Ambulance companies and emergency rooms in that area have little experience with pediatric cardiac emergencies. They can stabilize children and infants and then transfer them, usually by helicopter, to a metropolitan pediatric hospital.

Baby Epps's death was the result of a perfect storm. Because it was a weekend, the EMT and paramedic who were dispatched were relatively new; they had no practical experience with pediatric resuscitation and were unable to secure an airway and establish an intravenous line. They were instructed to transport the infant to the closest hospital. The ER there was closed on the weekends because of staffing shortages, so the ride to the nearest hospital with an open ER took three times longer. The skeleton staff at the more distant hospital did an admirable job of stabilizing Baby Epps and preparing him for a transfer to the children's hospital, but inclement weather was grounding the helicopter service. This was particularly unfortunate not only because an airlift would have been much faster, but also because the helicopter crew was experienced and better equipped to deal with pediatric emergencies.

Transfer proceeded by ambulance with a relatively inexperienced crew. All was well until severe arrhythmias popped up. The ambulance crew, as hard as they tried, could not treat the arrhythmias effectively. By the time Baby Epps finally arrived at Children's Hospital, the situation was hopeless. His tragic death may have been a blessing because the likelihood of severe damage to his brain during the long ride with a disorganized heart rhythm, and without an effective blood pressure, was very high.

Mr. and Mrs. Epps were devastated as was their family. One of their cousins was a personal injury attorney and encouraged them to have their case reviewed by his firm to determine if Baby Epps's care was negligent. They agreed to have the facts reviewed, which meant that Dr. Herr was delivered a summons for his records, engendering all the negative emotions that go with suggestions of malpractice. After several months, and a thorough review by a competent expert who opined that Dr. Herr's care was appropriate, the family elected not to pursue the case, to Dr. Herr's decided relief.

Mr. and Mrs. Epps were not dissuaded from having more children. They were counseled that Baby Epps's congenital abnormality was not likely to occur in subsequent offspring. But before they went ahead with their plans to get pregnant, they sold their farm and moved back into the city, a mile from the university's medical complex, vowing to never again be far away from high-quality medical assistance for their children, and for themselves.

COMMENTARY

As noted, Baby Epps's death occurred because of a constellation of bad luck. But, as with many complicated cases, there was an underlying issue that led directly to the misfortune. In this case, it was the lack of adequate medical facilities in a newly populated area, miles outside of two large cities.

The story of what went wrong in this rural area began years before. This sparsely populated community had two reasonably sized local hospitals. Given the simplicity of medicine in the mid-1900s, and with the support of the local community, the hospitals were more than adequate for the needs of the local citizenry and were never in financial trouble. Between government subsidies, charitable donations and fundraisers, and skilled management, the hospitals flourished.

Things changed rapidly in the 2000s. Medicine became a big business with astounding revenue generation and the potential for explosive growth. The reasons for this remarkable development have been discussed in previous stories, but much had to do with the entry of Medicare and guaranteed reimbursement, the development of new and expensive technology, and the aging of the Baby Boomers, which meant that millions of people would become heavy users of medical care.

With rising costs and the growing complexity of hospital and practice management, smaller institutions began to flounder. Community hospitals, so vital to the health of their local populations, could not keep up with the demand for more complex medical care. Newly minted subspecialists who wanted to establish high-tech programs were not always equipped or supported adequately to make their fledgling programs successful. After a few frustrating years and millions of dollars wasted, many of them folded.

As it became clear that smaller hospitals, try as they might, could not deliver the same quality and level of care as the university hospitals, most of them entered into agreements by which they would refer complex patients to major urban hospitals but keep simple procedures for themselves. That worked for a while until physicians, and especially those in large hospital systems, realized that they could safely carry out a variety of operations and procedures in stand-alone facilities. As these satellites proliferated, virtually free of regulation, small hospital revenues from common procedures like cataract extractions, joint replacement and colonoscopies, disappeared.

Another survival strategy used by floundering smaller hospitals was to associate with a famous medical center, giving rise to names such as the MD Anderson Cancer Center at Podunk General, or Cleveland Clinic Cardiac Care at Boondock Memorial. This expensive strategy was designed to persuade the public that their outcomes could be the same as if they were patients at the mothership. Missing, of course, were any details about what the relationship between the institutions meant to patients, and if outcomes improved with these affiliations. The massive amount of money spent on rebranding opportunities was not recouped by higher patient revenues. The advertisements attracted even sicker patients and a higher overhead.

Faced with shrinking revenue, but pressured by their neighborhoods to remain open, community hospitals had two alternatives. They could join a larger healthcare system as a "partner," or they could be bought out by a for-profit organization. Each had several disadvantages. Absorption into a large healthcare system meant surrender of governance and autonomy. Lip service was paid to continuing independence, but within a few years, that was all forgotten as the parent board imposed its will on the smaller members. Most importantly, the system administrators would decide where assets were allocated and how much technology each of the small hospitals would be allowed to keep or develop.

As disheartening as this might have been to local inhabitants who watched their home hospitals close, the disruption paled in comparison to the fate of those hospitals that were bought out by what would ultimately be called private equity. Here, the gambit was far more sinister. Although a few of the large corporations that made these purchases had good intentions, the vast majority never intended to preserve the hospitals they bought. As they had done in dozens of other industries, their plan was to load the small hospitals with debt, declare bankruptcy, peddle the assets, and then sell off most of the real estate.

The first part of the strategy was easy. Hospitals traditionally work on a very small operating margin, so it would take only a relatively short time to over-hire, over-purchase and overpay the executives before the hospital would be swimming in debt. The next maneuver was to begin to limit services, such as closing outpatient facilities, restricting the hours that the ER was open, and discontinuing inpatient services like obstetrics. The inevitable drop in revenue accelerated the hospital's descent into a hopeless financial situation that would ultimately result in closure and/or bankruptcy.

The extent of hospital plundering in the US is breathtaking. Hundreds of hospitals across the country have had to close or severely limit services, leaving people like Mr. and Mrs. Epps isolated and helpless. But the process has not been limited to "the sticks." Witness the closure of Hahnemann University Hospital in Philadelphia, one of the largest healthcare institutions and a thriving concern before it was bought out by a for-profit hospital chain. Inner-city patients in Philadelphia watched in horror as the physical plant literally fell apart without money allocated for routine maintenance. Patients had to bring in family members to care for them at night because there was virtually no chance of having a nurse, or even a patient care technician, answer a call for assistance. When the hospital finally closed, it was a catastrophe for patients, employees, house officers, medical students, and the community in general. Critically ill patients in intensive care units had to be transferred to hospitals, some miles away. Residents and staff scurried to find new positions in the region so as not to disrupt their families. Many landed at a hospital system south of Philadelphia, also run by a private equity firm, which didn't remain solvent for long. In that case, a private equity company had purchased two hospitals and promptly took out a loan for over a billion dollars, half of which was used to pay dividends to the CEO and their stockholders. They also sold the prime real estate on which the hospitals rested, forcing the already jeopardized institutions to pay rent. When the hospitals finally went under, thousands of patients and healthcare providers literally had nowhere to go.

How to restore credible care to "healthcare deserts" in rural areas or in the poor neighborhoods of big cities is not clear. One approach has been the development of "micro-hospitals," which house an emergency room and a few beds to keep patients stable until arrangements can be made for transfer to a real hospital. While sounding like a good idea, several details are missing such as what constitutes sufficient staffing, exactly how much equipment is required for medical stabilization, and who is going to absorb the cost of urgent medical transfers that are not easy and not cheap. With the growth of rural communities, one can easily anticipate overwhelming micro-hospitals with patients who have nowhere else to go in an emergency.

CONCLUSION

The public has the reasonable expectation that when they need medical care, it will be available and accessible. This is clearly not the case in a growing number of areas in the United States. We now have critical doctor shortages in primary care and in several key specialties. Trying to get an appointment with a psychiatrist, an endocrinologist, or a neurologist is an ordeal, with wait times of several months for new patients. Cardiologists, who are expected to deal with serious diseases, routinely have waiting lists that are weeks to months long. Fully half of the counties in the US have not one practicing cardiologist in their jurisdiction. One pundit remarked that if you can wait weeks to see a heart specialist, you probably didn't need the consultation in the first place. Conversely, if you really did need a prompt visit, you would likely be dead by the time you could get in.

Even with these outpatient care deficiencies, patients in need have had the bailout option of going to an urgent care center or, in more severe cases, to the local hospital emergency room. The former option may be realistic for non-serious conditions if the care provider is competent. Unfortunately, there are no assurances in that regard since urgent care centers can be staffed by almost anyone, including those with shoddy medical training. Hospital emergency rooms are packed with patients, many simply waiting to be triaged or admitted to hospital beds. In inner-city hospitals, 24-hour waits are not unheard of. In our region, hospitals go on "divert status" on a regular basis, which means that ambulances are directed not to bring patients to their ERs for lack of bed space. What happens to patients in that situation is unpredictable and scary.

Hospital bed availability is now in real jeopardy and, with proposed Medicaid cuts, things will only get much worse Acute care hospitals are under immense pressure, and few are now able to operate without a deficit. Those that remain open are crammed with patients. Given the lack of availability of primary care, and the aging of the population, patients are coming to the hospital sicker and needier than ever.

The idea that, in recent times, greedy, immoral, junk-bond billionaires would be able to strike the final blow and end the viability of so many US hospitals is infuriating. And yet they have moved into the medicine space with little or no oversight by state or federal regulators, or legislators. Not a single piece of federal legislation has been passed to prevent the pillaging of hospitals all over the country. The plunderers have been clever enough to adhere to the letter of current laws while placing millions of sick patients at risk.

As for community hospital acquisition by large health systems, while less threatening, this too has the potential to erode the quality and accessibility of healthcare. Big Medicine executives are several steps removed from the core business of medical care. Their job is to make money so they can continue to build palatial facilities and grow the bottom line. If that means consolidating or shutting off services to achieve an "economy of scale," so be it. Protests from their constituent medical staff, whom they regard as their employees, about their draconian decisions that negatively affect patient care are regarded as nothing more than annoying, if they are heard at all.

Hospital advertising has reached deafening levels. Even small hospitals spend millions to extoll their expertise and "cutting edge" technology, buttressed with in-name-only affiliations with famous medical centers. The irony is that the money spent on marketing nonsense, if used to hire nurses and ancillary staff, would help hospitals achieve the quality of care to which they say they aspire.

PATIENT ADVICE

What advice can we render to our vulnerable patients? Clearly, before deciding about where to live, especially in your sunset years, you will need an accurate idea of the quality and availability of urgent care in your area. Relying on outpatient clinics or the medical care that is available at your retirement facility is not adequate. It is inevitable that most of us, and our family members, will need to visit an emergency room at some point with the strong possibility of hospital admission. Where those facilities are, and how well they are staffed and maintained, is crucial information for the modern-day patient. So, before you start chasing your children and grandchildren across the country, keep in mind that medical care deserts are common and unlikely to be sufficiently populated anytime soon. Likewise, doctor shortages, especially in medical specialties, are becoming more common.

As a healthcare consumer, it is important to be critical. A little bit of investigation will reveal that most advertising claims are simply not supported by fact. When you are critically ill at some backwater medical institution, the Mayo brothers are *not* going to walk into your room and perform a miracle. Similarly, it isn't difficult to find a few former patients who are willing to be interviewed about their amazing experience at St. Elsewhere. Hospital advertisements overstate quality and expertise and do so without regulation or authentication.

As we have emphasized, a frank discussion with a person you trust is likely to yield a much better understanding of how best to position yourself to get the best possible medical care for yourself and your family over the long term.

Story 15: Affiliated Healthcare Professionals Are as Good as Doctors. Really?

"The greater the ignorance, the greater the dogmatism."
—Sir William Osler

NARRATIVE

Mrs. Hernandez was a pleasant 68-year-old Hispanic woman who, with her husband, immigrated to the United States and then established and ran a small grocery store in an inner-city neighborhood. To support their growing family, they worked hard for years, putting in long hours and enduring several holdups when they thought they were going to die. So, when their children were grown, they decided to reward themselves by selling the business and moving into a suburban retirement facility. They wanted to be close to their two pre-adolescent grandchildren while they were still healthy enough to enjoy them.

Mr. and Mrs. Hernandez were happy with their new life. To maintain their independence, they lived in a small cottage on the grounds of their retirement facility, yet still able to enjoy the facility's amenities. They grew particularly fond of playing bridge and cornhole with their neighbors and taking long walks on the hiking trails that surrounded the property.

Mr. and Mrs. Hernandez were in good health and worked hard to stay in shape. They pursued a prudent diet and avoided junk food to keep their weight under control. They both had borderline high blood pressure and cholesterol, but those problems were handled meticulously by the primary care physician who serviced their retirement facility. Mrs. Hernandez had a history of childhood seasonal asthma that infrequently recurred in adulthood, but she kept an inhaler in her purse and at her bedside in case of a rare recurrence.

All was well until Mrs. Hernandez developed a sore and swollen left calf. Local treatment didn't help so she consulted her primary care doctor. He told her he was worried that she might have a clot in one of the deep veins in her leg. He ordered a venous ultrasound study that was carried out at the local hospital the next day.

The test result was positive, showing a rather large clot in a main vein in her left thigh. The vascular specialist who read the test called Mrs. Hernandez's doctor with the results, and he immediately placed her on an oral blood thinner called Eliquis, also known as apixaban. This was a relatively new drug with an excellent efficacy and safety profile; it had supplanted warfarin (Coumadin) as the most prescribed oral blood thinner. Because of its rapid onset of action, Eliquis could be started on outpatients with the expectation that it would begin to work immediately. This obviated the need to be admitted to the hospital to receive intravenous medication until the effect of warfarin kicked in. Mrs. Hernandez was reassured that her insurance company would cover most of the cost and she would have to take it for only a few months until the clot resolved and the vein healed.

Things went well for Mrs. Hernandez. With continued local treatment and regular dosing with the blood thinner, the swelling and pain in her leg resolved within a few days. In a couple of weeks, she was back to her normal activity pattern. The only fly in the ointment was annoying nose bleeds, a known side-effect of Eliquis, which occurred every few days. Mrs. Hernandez found the bleeding disturbing but, on each occasion, she was able to stop the bleeding with a few minutes of nasal pressure. Nevertheless, she was eager to discontinue the drug not only because of the bleeding, but also because it was expensive. Contrary to what her doctor had assumed, her insurance company was paying only a small fraction of the monthly Eliquis bill of $700.

Mrs. Hernandez was told that the usual course of therapy for a serious deep vein thrombosis was at least three months and likely longer in patients like her who had a large clot. Mrs. Hernandez pushed back. She argued that with her excellent therapeutic result, a full three-month course might not be necessary. Her doctor reluctantly agreed to stop Eliquis after two months. Mrs. Hernandez was pleased with his decision, the outcome of her illness, her prompt return to full function, and the end of her nosebleeds.

About three months later, Mrs. Hernandez awoke in the middle of the night with shortness of breath. She sat up in bed gasping for air. She got to her inhaler, and used it without significant improvement. When her husband awoke, he was alarmed by her labored breathing and lack of response to the inhaler and insisted on a visit to the local hospital's emergency room. Mrs. Hernandez was reluctant, hoping that her shortness of breath would clear on its own. After several minutes, when things were no better, her husband finally prevailed and off they went to the ER.

On arrival, they were greeted by a clerk who, upon seeing Mrs. Hernandez in distress, called the triage nurse. With her husband in tow, Ms. Hernandez was ushered into the ER from the waiting area and placed on a stretcher. The nurse found that her vital signs were stable, but her blood oxygenation was on the low side. The nurse attached a nasal cannula, which caused a slight improvement in the oxygen saturation, and then told Mr. and Mrs. Hernandez that the doctor would be in to see her shortly.

A few minutes later, a young woman in a long white coat and a stethoscope in her pocket came through the curtain and introduced herself as Nurse Practitioner (NP) Antman. She explained that she was on duty in the emergency department and that she would be taking care of Mrs. Hernandez. Mr. and Mrs. Hernandez asked if they would eventually see a doctor and were reassured that the ER doctor on call was supervising her case.

NP Antman asked Mrs. Hernandez several questions about her symptoms and medical history and then examined her, listening to her heart and lungs. By this time, Mrs. Hernandez was feeling better and hoping that she had simply had a severe asthma attack, and that she wouldn't need to be admitted to the hospital.

NP Antman told Mrs. Hernandez that she was going to order a few relatively simple tests including bloodwork, a chest X-ray and an electrocardiogram. Mrs. Hernandez agreed as did her husband, and over the next hour, blood was drawn, an ECG was performed at bedside, and Mrs. Hernandez was brought to a radiology room off the ER, where she had the X-ray. Several minutes later, NP Antman reappeared and told Mrs. Hernandez that all her tests were fine. The most likely cause of her shortness of breath was an asthma attack. She explained it was not surprising that the inhaler hadn't worked since it was an old medication and possibly expired. Mrs. Hernandez was relieved and told NP Antman that she was eager to leave the emergency room. NP Antman said that before she could be discharged, the ER doctor on duty would have to review the case and agree with her assessment.

NP Antman began searching for her supervising physician and finally tracked him down as he waited on the phone to talk to a consultant about another case. After a cursory presentation, he agreed that Mrs. Hernandez could be discharged with the customary stipulation that she agree to be evaluated the next day by her primary care doctor.

NP Antman returned and delivered the good news to Hernandezes. She pointed out that her primary care doctor would likely provide her with a more effective and fresher inhaler for future episodes. She also told Mrs. Hernandez to return to the ER immediately if her symptoms recurred.

Mr. and Mrs. Hernandez were relieved and left the ER in good spirits. They arrived home, and after a light snack, retired to bed. Mr. Hernandez dropped off to sleep quickly but, given the excitement of the evening, Mrs. Hernandez decided to read for a while to settle her nerves.

Light was seeping through the bedroom curtains when Mr. Hernandez awoke to a scream and a crash. He scrambled out of bed and ran into the bathroom to find his wife lying unconscious on the floor. He couldn't rouse her and was unable to find a pulse. He called 911 and started to do CPR, taken over by the ambulance crew that arrived a few minutes later. The crew tried several drugs and also shocked her heart, but Mrs. Hernandez didn't respond. The crew continued CPR while transporting her to the same ER she had visited hours before. The doctor who had allowed her to be discharged but had never met her declared Mrs. Hernandez dead on arrival.

CASE EXPLANATION

Because of the circumstances of her death, Mrs. Hernandez's family requested an autopsy. Fortunately, the local coroner agreed so they didn't have to pay a large fee. The autopsy was carried out the next day so as not to interfere with funeral plans. The post-mortem findings were straightforward. Mrs. Hernandez had died from a massive pulmonary embolism. A large clot had re-developed in her legs and traveled to her heart and out into the pulmonary arteries, which carry blood to the lungs for oxygenation. The huge clot, referred to as a saddle embolus, had closed off all blood flow to the lungs making oxygenation impossible. This explained Mrs. Hernandez's collapse and cardiac arrest, and the inability to resuscitate her. The autopsy also found clots in smaller lung vessels that were not as fresh and were likely responsible for her first episode of shortness of breath that brought her to the ER the day before.

Let's return to the fateful ER visit that occurred a few hours before her death. Mrs. Hernandez was evaluated by a young and inexperienced nurse practitioner. She had been working in the ER only a few weeks and had only one short ER rotation during her clinical training. Mrs. Hernandez was never seen or examined by the ER physician who was supposed to be supervising the nurse practitioner. If he had, important facts might have been uncovered and a correct diagnosis made, saving her life.

Most importantly, NP Antman did not elicit Mrs. Hernandez's history of a deep vein thrombosis, which had been diagnosed five months earlier. She hadn't asked about recent illnesses, and Mrs. Hernandez either forgot to bring it up or didn't think that a clot in her leg was relevant to what was being called an asthma attack. Even worse, NP Antman didn't take the time to retrieve Mrs. Hernandez's hospital records. If she had, she would have seen a positive venous ultrasound that had led to the decision to prescribe a systemic anticoagulant. She also might have learned that Mrs. Hernandez, because of nosebleeds and cost, had insisted on coming off the anticoagulant before finishing a full three months of treatment, rendering her particularly susceptible to a clot recurrence.

Pulmonary embolism is a common cause of death in elderly people. It is frequently not suspected pre-mortem but when it is, the diagnosis is straightforward. First, there is a blood test called a D-dimer level that indicates ongoing thrombosis or clotting somewhere in the body. A CAT scan of the chest, a very available and easy test, would have been diagnostic in Mrs. Hernandez's case, revealing clot in the pulmonary vasculature. Anticoagulation would have been started in the ER with the strong probability that further embolization and death would have been prevented. If the clot at that point was large, Mrs. Hernandez may have been a candidate for intravenous medication to dissolve the clot, or a catheter procedure to extract it.

None of that mattered in the Hernandez case, because the diagnosis was missed entirely. What had probably been a smaller clot that caused the first milder episode was not diagnosed and treated. Tragically, that set the stage for a second, much larger clot to travel to the lungs and precipitate a total circulatory collapse with no hope of resuscitation.

Mrs. Hernandez's history of asthma was what medical people refer to as a "red herring." It was a distraction that made it easier for NP Antman and her supervising doctor to reach an incorrect diagnosis. Mrs. Hernandez had not responded to the inhaler and had never had an asthma attack that awakened her from sleep. These were important historical facts that a seasoned clinician would have elicited and then considered in forming a differential diagnosis, or a list of the things that might have been causing Mrs. Hernandez's shortness of breath. From that list, he or she would have ordered appropriate testing to focus on the most likely diagnosis. The inexperienced NP Antman had no ability to consider various possibilities or the means to consider or reject them.

COMMENTARY

Doctors spend years in training for a good reason. It is only with a well-developed knowledge of the basic sciences, careful tutelage by learned mentors, and extensive bedside experience that a student can develop into a physician capable of making a correct diagnosis and saving a life. It is why we say that doctors "practice" medicine. We are constantly honing our skills, and getting wiser is possible only with a strong knowledge base garnered during intensive medical school study and house officer training.

To expect a nurse with only weeks of classroom instruction and a few months of practitioner training and experience to have the same reflexes and instincts as a seasoned clinician would be humorous were it not so tragic. The willingness of patients to accept a substitute points out how difficult it is for the public to judge the quality and expertise of practitioners.

NP Antman was hired out of her training specifically to see patients in one of the most complicated areas of the hospital, the emergency room. Those of us who have worked there know how daunting it is to evaluate sick patients you don't know in the pressure cooker of an ER. The complexity of the job explains why ER doctors have high rates of suicide, job dissatisfaction, and early retirement.

Not only were NP Antman's skills inadequate but so was the amount of oversight. Her supervising ER physician never saw Mrs. Hernandez because he didn't have the time and he wasn't expected to do so. He never analyzed the case in detail or made suggestions about various possible diagnoses or appropriate diagnostic tests. Instead, while on the phone and distracted, he listened for a couple of minutes to NP Antman's presentation, looked over the results of the inappropriate tests she had ordered, and agreed with her plan to attribute Mrs. Hernandez's symptoms to asthma and discharge her.

NP Antman erred several times during her bedside evaluation of Mrs. Hernandez. If NP Antman had asked, Mrs. Hernandez would have told her that almost all her asthma attacks occurred during exertion and never at rest. She also would have learned that Mrs. Hernandez's asthma was seasonal and unlikely to occur in the winter months. But perhaps the most egregious error was not taking a complete past medical history. Mr. and Mrs. Hernandez didn't tell NP Antman that she had a recent deep vein thrombosis, probably because they didn't know why it might be related to shortness of breath. Depending on elderly patients to volunteer key information is another example of clinical naivete.

NP Antman compounded her history-taking error by not reviewing Mrs. Hernandez's electronic medical record. The advent of the EMR is both a help and a hindrance in this regard. Unlike the "old days" of paper records when someone had to fetch charts from the remote file room, Mrs. Hernandez's recent test results were easily accessible on a computer terminal. However, to bring up and review those records electronically requires precious doctor time, sifting through what might be hundreds of pages of documents to finally discover a relevant test result. In the world of "fast medicine" in which doctors are expected to turn ER beds over and see dozens of patients in an impossibly short time, accessing old records by any method is all too commonly ignored.

The truth is that affiliated healthcare professionals or physician extenders are enormously valuable people. When properly trained and supervised, they are a marvelous addition to the healthcare team, saving enormous amounts of time for physicians. They can assist with various procedures and in many cases, become nearly as technically proficient as physicians themselves. They can spend more time with patients and families than doctors and establish profound therapeutic relationships. They are eager to learn and to expand their fund of knowledge because they appreciate that they will become better practitioners only if someone teaches them. Physician extenders I have had the good fortune to supervise have become terrific colleagues, avidly seeking to be mentored and supervised to evolve into even better practitioners.

Problems arise when they, or their professional society representatives, insist on independent practice such as when there is no doctor in residence, or, as in Mrs. Hernandez's case, a doctor is in the vicinity to review cases and approve NP decisions. Independent practice in these situations is unacceptable, in my opinion. In most such cases, NP notes and orders are rubber-stamped and there is little to no time for bedside teaching and hands-on instruction. If physician assistants are making mistakes, they will never be corrected by signing their charts, and their level of care never elevated. Compounding the problem is the new idea of using physician extenders to care for patients using telemedicine. The recent and highly publicized case of a limb amputation caused by inadequate remote care of a patient with vascular disease by a poorly supervised physician's assistant will have the effect of making telemedicine, a fundamentally good idea, less accessible for everyone.

How did we allow things to get to this point? It happened for the simple reason that we don't have enough doctors to take care of all the patients who need us. Instead of correcting the problem by increasing doctor supply, for example, by loosening ridiculous limitations on the licensing of immigrant physicians, we have decided to permit independent practice by physician extenders, many of whom are unaware of their shortcomings. Their professional organizations have made the situation worse by exerting political pressure to gain more freedom for their members. They persuade ignorant legislators to loosen regulations on NPs by citing how difficult it is for so many patients to access care, deliberately ignoring the huge differences in expertise and quality between doctors and NPs. These organizations have even resorted to television commercials that advise patients to "choose a nurse practitioner [over a doctor]." They encourage their members to obtain PhDs in nursing so patients can call them "doctor." They have pushed hard to rename physician assistants as "physician associates" to elevate their status. With all this obfuscation, patients are uninformed about the expertise of the person taking responsibility for their care, and, in some settings like the ER, literally making life and death decisions.

CONCLUSION

Medicine is a complicated business, a fact that is underappreciated by the lay public. They have been brainwashed by TV-show drivel wherein "geniuses" in white coats cure patients with ease while pursuing their latest romantic relationships. It takes years of education and practice to produce a seasoned clinician. As we have discussed, it is an agonizing process. Imagine a physician's consternation when, despite all the blood, sweat, tears and money they spent to hone their medical skills, they are treated like fungible pawns by superiors and legislators who have no comprehension of what they do.

In their naïvete, these non-practicing authoritarians believe they can shortcut the process of physician development and manufacture drones who will function just as well as doctors and for a much lower salary. The notion is absurd, but unfortunately it has become popularized to the point that even the automatons themselves believe it. It doesn't take much effort to convince foolish and self-serving legislators to pass laws perpetuating the insanity, and before you can blink, patients adjust and become accustomed to a wholly reduced quality of medical care.

The real crime is that the idea of training and hiring doctor assistants is brilliant. Every doctor knows how valuable a good nurse can be. Elevating such people to practitioner status makes sense. When incorporated into a well-oiled medical care delivery machine, the result is greatly enhanced patient care. We can only hope for continued development of the "team" concept in which all the players know and embrace their role. Mechanisms must be put into place whereby our assistants are correctly and constantly supervised by physicians who feel comfortable in that role and are willing to take the time to do it right.

PATIENT ADVICE

Once again, physicians depend on their professional organizations to exert whatever influence remains to them to preserve the highest quality of care. But these initiatives will succeed only if fully supported by informed and proactive patients who are willing to lobby politicians and legislators to enact regulations that control what physician assistants and nurse practitioners can and cannot do in specific clinical settings.

In the meantime, the message is clear: don't settle for a physician replacement in any important healthcare interaction unless you are convinced that she or he is properly trained and closely supervised. Don't be afraid to ask who is making the decisions about how your healthcare is conducted, and who is responsible for the consequences. Only be afraid if you get no answer or one you don't want to hear.

Story 16: Research Data and How to Manipulate Them

"There are lies, damned lies, and statistics."
—Attributed to Benjamin Disraeli

NARRATIVE

Mr. Quinn was a 58-year-old African American man in big trouble. In his youth and early adulthood, he hadn't taken very good care of himself. He smoked three packs of cigarettes a day, had at least one six-pack of beer a day, ate a lot of junk food, and these bad habits, along with a heavy family history of stroke and heart attack, predisposed him to severe coronary artery disease. He had already suffered three heart attacks and had been hospitalized several times with heart failure with fluid backing up into his lungs so severely that he needed to be on a ventilator for several days.

His doctor, who practiced at a large and prestigious university medical center not far from Mr. Quinn's home, had implanted a cardiac defibrillator and a special pacemaker to synchronize his cardiac chambers and maximize his cardiac output, and had prescribed ten different drugs for various cardiac indications, but Mr. Quinn was not getting better. He was told that he would have been considered for a heart transplant except for his severe lung disease, acquired not only because of his smoking habit but also by working in a coal mine for several years when he was younger. He declined a left ventricular assist device, an electrical pump that would augment his cardiac function because he didn't want to carry a pump around for the rest of his life. He was unable to enjoy any part of his life, not even his grandchildren whom he adored.

To supplement Mr. Quinn's modest disability income, Mrs. Quinn worked across town in a small hospital's cafeteria. One winter afternoon, she returned from work, excited to tell her husband that a doctor at her hospital, during a radio interview, reported some amazing results with an experimental treatment called stem cell therapy. She didn't know the details, but she had copied down the telephone number for patients to call if they were interested in becoming a research subject. From the description on the radio, it sounded as if her husband would be a perfect candidate for the trial.

Initially, Mr. Quinn was reluctant. He was depressed and had given up hope that he would ever feel better and return to normal activity, but he told his family that he didn't want to be a "guinea pig." Mrs. Quinn was a patient person, and over the next several days, she and their children reminded him of the research opportunity, encouraging him to at least talk to the doctor in charge of the trial. Her hospital was abuzz with information about the project, with the hospital leadership hoping that the publicity surrounding it would attract patients and money they sorely needed to stay open.

Mr. Quinn began to consider the idea but insisted on first conferring with his cardiologist, a heart failure specialist at the university hospital. At his next monthly visit, he asked if stem cell therapy of the heart was a good idea. The cardiologist said it was too early to tell. The theory of infusing undifferentiated cells into the heart and hoping they would mature into healthy heart cells to strength heart function was reasonable, but it had to be tested in rigorous clinical trials. Mr. Quinn asked if the clinical trial at his wife's hospital could be an option. His cardiologist hadn't heard of the trial, the company or the doctors who were conducting the study, so he couldn't or perhaps wouldn't say. He did tell Mr. Quinn to be careful when considering new treatments that hadn't been proven.

Mr. Quinn discussed the situation again with his wife and two daughters at their Sunday dinner. All three of them encouraged him to relent, and reluctantly he did. The next morning, he called and made an appointment with Dr. Vijay at Community Hospital. During the phone call, he was asked several questions about his insurance and past medical history, and he was instructed to come in with his medical records, especially those related to his cardiac condition.

Dr. Vijay's office was well-appointed and the receptionist friendly. Mr. and Mrs. Quinn were ushered into an examination room, where they met a research nurse. She asked several questions, performed a perfunctory examination on Mr. Quinn, and then gathered up his medical records and said that Dr. Vijay would be in soon. A few minutes later, Dr. Vijay appeared in a starched white coat and, with a beaming smile, welcomed the Quinns to his cardiology practice.

Dr. Vijay sat across from Mr. and Mrs. Quinn and over the next several minutes asked questions about Mr. Quinn's clinical situation and previous treatments. He then described what the stem cell treatment was all about. Information gathered in "pre-clinical" studies had been promising. Researchers in Japan and China had shown that infusing stem cells into animals that had sustained heart damage from mechanical coronary artery occlusion had greatly improved heart function within weeks, returning it almost back to normal. Importantly, the infusions were not associated with any major side effects.

The company that invented the stem cells was planning a large randomized clinical study in Asia but was conducting a small, exploratory open-label trial in the US. That meant that all the patients who entered the trial would get stem cells, and none would receive placebo. The company had targeted a few clinical sites, and Community Hospital was one of them. They were about half-way through their first-in-human study and things were going very well. Patients hadn't experienced any major side effects, and several had reported a remarkable improvement in their symptoms. Dr. Vijay said it was too soon to conclude whether the stem cells had improved cardiac function or life expectancy. However, he was optimistic that the treatment would not only be effective but would "revolutionize" the treatment of patients who had heart attacks and scarring in the heart, prolonging the lives of heart failure victims, and effectively making heart transplants and assist devices obsolete.

Dr. Vijay explained how the drug would be given and all the possible side effects, again emphasizing that so far there had been no major problems. The stem cells would be harvested from anonymous donors who had a genetic profile like Mr. Quinn's, would be purchased by the hospital and supplied for free. Mr. Quinn would be responsible only for the cost of the infusions. Since it was considered an experimental therapy, Mr. Quinn's insurance company would likely not reimburse him for the $5000 fee for each of the six infusions.

Mr. and Mrs. Quinn were encouraged but concerned about the costs. They had saved money for retirement, and they had tried hard not to tap into those funds. But after they discussed it briefly among the family, they agreed they had little choice but to go forward. Mr. Quinn was only getting worse by the day.

The Quinns eventually signed the several consent forms and documents that would permit entry into the study. Mr. Quinn was given slips to have lab work and few other tests, including a DNA test. Once they had a stem cell match, he would have screening studies, including an echocardiogram to measure cardiac function. They would also test to see how far he could walk in six minutes, and he would fill out a detailed health questionnaire. Unfortunately, the Quinns would have to pay out of pocket for all the qualifying tests.

As soon as all of that was completed, and provided that the results met the entry criteria, Dr. Vijay would start the treatments, consisting of a thirty-minute intravenous infusion under observation in a procedure room in his office suite. A nurse would be present during the infusion in case of an adverse reaction, the most common of which was irritation at the infusion site and an allergic rash, neither of which was expected to be severe or dangerous. Mr. Quinn would receive six monthly treatments followed by a repeat set of tests to determine if the drug had worked to improve his symptoms, his stamina and his cardiac function.

With all the qualifying tests completed, the Quinn family waited anxiously for the study approval to come through. When Dr. Vijay's office called to deliver the good news of his acceptance into the study, they celebrated with a family dinner and a bottle of low-alcohol champagne. They toasted to Mr. Quinn's future good health and a new lease on his life.

Mr. Quinn's first treatment went well. He had no side effects from the infusions and was happy with the quality of care he received from the research staff. He decided to transfer all of his cardiology care to Dr. Vijay, who was delighted to take him on as a patient, agreeing heartily that there was no need for Mr. Quinn to see two cardiologists with the same expertise in treating heart failure.

By the time Mr. Quinn finished his sixth infusion, he was feeling much improved. His wife noticed that he was in a better mood. He was able to do chores around the house and spend time chasing his grandchildren. He was even able to do a little yard work and carry groceries for his wife, tasks that months before were impossible. Mr. Quinn's six-minute walk distance and his quality-of-life scores had nearly doubled compared to his pre-treatment values. The echocardiograms that were performed to objectively quantify his cardiac function had been submitted to the core laboratory in China for interpretation and the results were not yet available for review. Dr. Vijay said he was sure they would show improvement, given Mr. Quinn's remarkable functional gains.

Mr. Quinn was enormously grateful to Dr. Vijay, who was delighted by the results. Dr. Vijay told Mr. Quinn that if all went well, he might be a candidate for a long-term extension study during which he could receive less frequent but regular stem cell infusions to sustain the benefit he had already derived.

Things began to unravel a few months later when the prestigious cardiology journal that had published the article reporting the animal experiment results on which the stem cell program was based forced the authors to retract their article. One of the assistants at the laboratory in China that had conducted the experiments had gone to the dean of his medical school and alleged that the principal investigator had fabricated the data. His allegations were eventually substantiated, and the researcher was forced to resign in disgrace.

Given the magnitude of the scandal, and since the fraudulent article was the basis for the clinical trials in progress and those planned, the media zeroed in on the story. The whistleblower was interviewed on every primetime news outlet in the US. The FDA, which had granted an investigational license to the stem cell manufacturer to administer the drug in the US, withdrew its approval and ordered all the investigative sites to stop the treatments and discontinue patient enrollment. Most importantly, they were mandated to brief each patient in the trial, to make them aware of the strong possibility that the stem cell therapy didn't work and might even have undisclosed toxicity. Mr. Quinn received a certified letter from Dr. Vijay's office apprising him that the study had closed and encouraging him to make an appointment with the doctor to discuss next steps.

Mr. and Mrs. Quinn were upset and anxious for their next visit with Dr. Vijay. They were angry to have been entered into a clinical trial that had been based on tainted data and to have paid dearly out of their retirement funds for six stem cell infusions not supported by science. Not only that, but the gains Mr. Quinn had achieved in function were waning rapidly; he felt as if he was back where he was before he started the treatments.

When they arrived at Dr. Vijay's office for Mr. Quinn's appointment, they were told that the doctor had an emergency and that they would be seen by his nurse practitioner. Though disappointed, they agreed and were placed in an examination room where they waited for over an hour. When the harried nurse practitioner finally appeared, they bombarded her with questions about the study termination and the implications for Mr. Quinn's care. She admitted she didn't have much new information to relate to them, except that Mr. Quinn's other care would continue as before, including all the medications he had been prescribed by his first heart failure specialist.

Mr. Quinn asked for a refund for the $30,000 he had paid out of pocket for a worthless treatment. He was told he would have to take that up with the billing office, conversations that subsequently went nowhere. Mrs. Quinn wanted to know the results of the echocardiograms that had been carried out before and after Mr. Quinn's treatment to quantify anticipated improvement in cardiac function. Those results were still not in hand, according to the nurse practitioner. In fact, the company that had been conducting the study had closed its doors and was not returning phone calls or emails from any of the US investigators.

Mr. and Mrs. Quinn left the office disgruntled and depressed. They decided that Mr. Quinn should discontinue care with Dr. Vijay and return to his former heart failure cardiologist, who was happy to take him back. The doctor was sympathetic and told Mr. and Mrs. Quinn that he had heard about the trial's problems and had not been surprised. Other stem cell trials had also failed, and the entire area of research was in turmoil. He said that before human research could resume, a substantial amount of legitimate research would be needed to prove the value of infusing undifferentiated cells into any organ with the hope of restoring function. When asked why he had not been more forceful in his recommendations about avoiding stem cell therapy, the doctor admitted that physicians, given the uncertainties of medicine, are loathe to speak badly about colleagues. In this case, he admitted that not speaking up was his mistake.

Since the results of the echocardiograms that were carried out in the study were not available, Mr. Quinn had another echocardiogram at the office. The couple was disappointed to learn that his cardiac function was about the same as it was a year ago, before he had the stem cell infusions. The cardiologist tried to lessen the blow by simplifying Mr. Quinn's medical program and setting up a less intensive follow-up schedule to save the Quinns as much of their remaining retirement dollars as possible.

CASE EXPLANATION

Mr. Quinn suffered from a condition called ischemic cardiomyopathy. Each of his previous heart attacks had been caused by severe coronary artery disease. When the heart is deprived of adequate blood flow, heart cells die and are replaced by scars that do not contract. If the size of the scar tissue is substantial, cardiac function declines to the point at which the walls of the heart weaken and heart failure develops. That means that fluid begins to accumulate in the lungs and in the lower extremities, and the patient develops shortness of breath and diminished energy. Several measures can be taken to improve symptoms, such as diuretics that prompt a loss of excess fluid, but none of them are curative and few of them improve cardiac function.

Despite an array of treatments, Mr. Quinn was in dire straits. He was not a candidate for transplantation or for other advanced measures to improve pump function. In desperation, he had agreed to participate in a widely advertised research program that was not supported by good science. How did an ineffective therapy progress to human experimentation? A major reason was the medical community's enthusiasm for the concept, based on the knowledge that multi-potential embryonic cells could, under the correct circumstances and stimulation, differentiate into functioning cells in the organs into which they were injected. Also, there was little downside since the treatments had few known side effects. The idea of regenerating cardiac tissue was so compelling that eagerness outstripped science and several experiments were launched prematurely.

The methods that were used in Mr. Quinn's case were the least likely to meet with success. The cells that were infused were from matched donors. The best chance of a "take" comes with cells harvested from the patient's own bone marrow, a taxing procedure that Mr. Quinn may not have tolerated and likely would have declined. In addition, the cells for Mr. Quinn were infused through a peripheral vein. Direct placement of stem cells into the heart during cardiac surgery or through a catheter in the coronary artery increases the density of cells delivered to the areas where they are needed, improving the chances of a good outcome.

Not only was the scientific basis for the stem cell trial weak, but so was the experimental design. First, in this first-in-human study, there was no control group. Though that meant that all the patients would receive active therapy, and no one would be left out, exact quantification of efficacy and safety of a new treatment without a simultaneous placebo control group is impossible. The primary endpoint of the study was patient symptoms and their ability to walk a distance. Both tests are subject to substantial bias. Since the patients knew they received active treatment, they wanted to improve. The placebo effect in this situation can be quite strong and mimic or obscure a true treatment benefit. Mr. Quinn felt better for a while and convinced himself to walk further, but objective proof of mechanical improvement by echocardiography, to his disappointment, was lacking and his gains were fleeting.

Dr. Vijay practiced at Community Hospital, a small institution without a substantial research reputation or portfolio. But advancing science was not Dr. Vijay's primary mission. His group wanted to make money, so they searched for projects that had substantial revenue potential. They advertised their research projects heavily in the media, playing on the emotions of end-stage patients who needed hope. Also, by selecting protocols that featured the need for drug injections, they were able to feed their own infusion center and charge the patient directly for that service. That revenue was several-fold what they paid the Chinese company for worthless stem cells, insuring a healthy profit for each subject enrolled.

Was it a coincidence that Dr. Vijay was not present at Mr. Quinn's follow-up visit, or did he not want to face the angry couple who had been duped into enrolling in a meaningless trial? And what of the lack of availability of the one test result that was intended to prove conclusively that the stem cells had improved cardiac function, the echocardiogram?

Despite returning to the competent care of the university heart failure service, Mr. Quinn would die a year later. He was admitted many times over his final months for treatments to relieve the load on his heart and to dry out his lungs and legs, which had become congested with fluids. Despite best efforts, his heart finally gave out and he passed away quietly with his family at his bedside.

COMMENTARY

Research is the engine that drives medical care. Every drug and every device used in contemporary practice was developed in elaborate research programs. These begin at the bench, where astute scientists search diligently for new ways to treat disease. Some of these individuals reside in academia, but many are pharmaceutical and device company employees. Their full-time job is to discover, develop, investigate and file for the approval of new chemical or device entities. By most metrics, they have been enormously successful. We have multiplied the number of treatment options for common as well as rare diseases, including congestive heart failure, with marked improvement in important outcomes like death, hospitalizations and quality of life.

As in other areas of medicine, the potential for large revenue generation has changed the focus of clinical research. Small biotech companies, backed by venture capital, have sprung up with the goal of finding treatments for relatively rare diseases, hoping that unmet medical need would justify a huge price tag for their remedies. Big Pharma has become obsessed with discovering "blockbuster" drugs with the potential to generate billions of dollars in revenue over a relatively short period of patent life. Large academic medical centers compete for federal funding that provides billions of dollars of overhead for their grand institutions, money that could instead be spent funding worthy grant proposals These university centers also dream of patenting the discoveries of their faculty and reaping millions if not billions of dollars for their already bloated endowments. And healthcare providers like Dr. Vijay who are not at all interested in science have figured out how to make money by enrolling patients in clinical trials that may be poorly conceived or have little scientific value.

Another "side-effect" of the commercialization of research is cheating. With so much to gain from a successful research program, such as attracting grant or venture capital money, it shouldn't be surprising that we have seen a sharp uptick in the number of fraudulent research projects which, after their exposure, force the authors to retract the papers. Thousands of articles are taken back by scientists for various reasons, but cheating is at the top of the list. We have witnessed the retraction of highly publicized research papers, and in the worst case, removal of approved drugs and devices from the market because of cheating during the conduct of trials that supported regulatory approval. Unfortunately, we have no idea how often cheating occurs on a smaller scale, for example, hiding or altering an essential finding. The direst aspect is that a fraudulent research result, given the possibility of wide dissemination at professional society meetings and through social media, can sidetrack an important therapeutic area and in some cases be its death knell.

Recently we have seen the beginnings of government intrusion into the publication process, not only by denying funding of grants that conservatives consider unacceptable, but also by tasking journal editors with ensuring "balanced" viewpoints for controversial issues. Government interference with the medical scientific process should send a chill down the spine of anyone who values truth in science.

Actual flat-out cheating in research, as despicable as it is, is a smaller problem than data manipulation. Consider the investigator who, disappointed with her results, decides to change the statistical analysis methods just enough to make the result positive. Or the researcher who knowingly tilts the method of patient recruitment to enroll a population more likely to respond to the new drug or device. Some of these manipulations may not even be intentional. Journals that publish important research results are ordinarily not privy to the raw data that generated the submitted manuscript. Researchers are not compelled to submit those data, and it is usually so voluminous that journal editors and reviewers, who work for nothing, would never be able to wade through the mountains of information. Many times, it is not until the rigorous review of a regulatory submission for marketing approval, that sleight of hand or honest analysis mistakes are discovered by full-time reviewers.

I was taught early in my training to "beware of the tyranny of small numbers." Not only do studies need to be properly designed and interpreted, but they also need to be adequately sized. This is especially true when the disease in question is highly prevalent. With millions of Americans manifesting coronary artery disease every year, it seems ridiculous to rely on studies of dozens or even hundreds of patients subjected to a new drug or procedure. And yet, that is exactly what has happened in many disease states such as congestive heart failure. Inadequately powered studies increase the risk of selection bias and inadvertent confounding that render the results uninterpretable at best and invalid at worst. Investigators and funding agencies and regulators have finally begun to understand how important the powering of a trial is to the proper interpretation of its results.

However, second- and third-rate journals, eager to attract new study results, are fertile ground for publishing nonsensical papers that attract media attention because of their "importance to the public." These journals further bastardize the research process by charging exorbitant publication fees that discourage young investigators who do not have sufficient funding to carry out original research, let alone pay to get their findings into print. The average fee to publish a peer-reviewed paper in an "open access" journal, which allows non-subscribers to access manuscripts for free, is more than $3000.

To attract attention to a new finding, one frequently used ploy is to ignore the fact that an experiment found no difference in the overall patient population that was studied, and to move on to consider sub-groups with the hope of finding anybody who might benefit from the new therapy. While such an exercise may be hypothesis generating, it is never definitive. It does, however, provide talking points for authors eager to attract media attention to their research. Another deceptive tactic is to report a relative rather than an absolute risk reduction. For example, if a new treatment reduced symptoms in three treated subjects compared to five in a placebo group, the authors would could message a lofty forty percent relative treatment effect, when in reality an absolute difference of two would more likely be the play of chance.

None of these issues with clinical research are as maddening as the intentionally misleading "clinical studies" that are used to support worthless healthcare products. Remember that individual testimonies are all that is required for a homeopathic drug to be advertised and sold, and yet the snake oil purveyors repeatedly refer to "clinical studies" or "published research" in their TV commercials to swindle the public. While these wild claims are being made, the small print at the bottom of the screen, if you can see it, will specify that what is being advertised has never been shown to prevent or treat any disease.

Headline news frequently reports the results of "important clinical trials" that yield fantastic results. It is rare for any of those stories to contain actual study methods or result data. Take, for example, a recent study, which concluded that multivitamins slow aging. From the topline results, I would have assumed that the study found that people who take multivitamins have a longer life expectancy. The real story, however, is that researchers, using undisclosed methods, found that genes aged slower in people who took one of a variety of vitamins, at various doses. While the findings were interesting and worthy of further investigation, they were far from definitive enough to warrant news coverage.

Stem cell treatments and infusions of platelet-rich plasma have become popular ways to scam the public. The idea is to implant cells that can differentiate into the target tissue type and repair damaged organs. They have been touted to treat a wide variety of diseases with little or no evidence of benefit. One of the most popular is the injection of stem cells into joints to treat osteoarthritis. In media ads, doctors who claim to be orthopedic surgeons describe the amazing benefits of these treatments, including avoidance of joint replacement surgery. These "physicians" prey on the elderly who are plagued with severe joint pain and young athletes who wish to continue their careers, despite serious injuries. Charging large fees for worthless treatments not covered by insurance is an unforgivable violation of their oath. Exactly why government regulators who are charged with protecting citizens permit this kind of skullduggery is a mystery and a scandal. Even more frightening is that the current Secretary of Health and Human Services has signaled his intention to loosen regulation of stem cell treatment because, with absolutely no expertise or evidence, he believes in its effectiveness and safety.

As if to throw gasoline on the fire, witless politicians have been petitioned by patient advocates to pass legislation allowing desperate individuals to gain access to drugs that are under investigation but not yet fully approved by regulatory agencies. The so-called "right to try" movement is predicated on the idea that patients on the verge of death shouldn't have to wait until new drugs have been thoroughly vetted because they have nothing to lose. This concept reveals an incredible naivete about the drug approval process. For every drug that is found to be safe and effective, scores of new agents fall short, either because of unacceptable toxicity, inadequate efficacy or both. Unapproved drugs have insufficient information regarding dosing and drug interactions that make their early adoption highly hazardous. Public advocacy of a bizarre idea such as "right to try" also reflects the lack of transparency in the drug development business. Corporations maintain strict secrecy about their research programs as they struggle to gain an advantage over competitors, a situation that further ripens the possibilities of behind-the-scenes data manipulation.

Our government hasn't finished ruining American medical research. They have now chosen to revoke funding for hundreds of important projects because of their determination to squash anything that smells of transgenderism or vaccine advocacy. University research programs are scaling back, and foreign governments are actively recruiting American investigators who have lost their federal funding. Interference of this kind in medical research will have dire consequences, which will reverberate for many years to come.

CONCLUSION

The prognosis for heart failure is worse than for most forms of cancer. So the search for more effective therapies, including stem cell replacement, will continue, as it should. This will necessarily require early-phase trials in which there can be no guarantee of clinical benefit. But that is not Mr. Quinn's story. His treatment failed because a scientist cheated, and a greedy doctor wanted to make more money. Perpetration of fraudulent or misleading research information is truly frightening because it places all of us at the mercy of unprincipled scientists and marketeers who derail good medical care in the name of profit. Regulatory bodies, like the FDA, protect us against the most egregious charlatans, but the medical enterprise is so vast, and the FDA budget so small, that opportunities for mischief abound. The withdrawal or recall of faulty drugs and devices occurs with alarming frequency. Some of this is unavoidable. Complex medical research is hard, and mistakes are inevitable. But we need to do away with exaggerations of efficacy and dismissal of toxicity that have become commonplace, especially in direct-to-consumer medical advertising. Likewise, we need to protect against bias in the many competitive aspects of academic medicine such as grant review, peer review of manuscripts and scientific meeting abstracts, and faculty governance and promotion. Likewise, we need to advocate for academic freedom and efforts to keep the United States at the forefront of medical research. Our patients deserve no less.

PATIENT ADVICE

Rushing to new and relatively unproven treatments has always been a hazard, prompting the legendary clinician, Sir William Osler, to paraphrase Trousseau's admonition, "use the new drugs now, while they still work." The patient public needs to be vigilant and to maintain healthy skepticism about any new treatment, particularly those endorsed by a celebrity during a Super Bowl. It should not be a surprise that patients are searching for alternative treatments when mainstream therapies are costly and their health insurance inadequate. Putting those issues right would be another important way of quelling the rise of questionable or outright worthless treatments.

As always, paramount is a strong line of communication with a knowledgeable and honest healthcare provider who is willing to answer questions and to provide learned advice about all remedies, unbiased by his or her professional relationships or standing or financial interests. We must depend on these good practitioners to counsel patients no matter how difficult the message, rather than remaining quiet and tacitly allowing unprincipled colleagues to prey on unwitting and suffering patients.

Story 17: Diversity and Inclusion: Do We Need a VP or a Dean for That?

"When we're talking about diversity, it is not a box to check. It is a reality that should be deeply felt and valued by all of us." —Ava DuVernay

NARRATIVE

Ms. Engle was a 55-year-old African American woman who worked at Upstate College as a vice-dean for admissions. She was single and never married and lived in a quiet neighborhood just a half mile from the campus. Her four siblings lived in a nearby city, and she enjoyed visiting them and playing the good aunt to their children. She had a dog and a cat that she loved dearly, and a supportive network of friends. By all accounts, her life was rich.

Ms. Engle was proud to be an African American and participated in several organizations that promoted racial minorities. Her public relations job at Upstate College included promoting diversity among the student body, a daunting task, given the relatively small number of African Americans and other minorities who applied for admission and were admitted to the undergraduate student body.

As part of her commitment to diversity, Ms. Engle actively sought out minority service providers. To support their businesses, she preferred to hire Black electricians, plumbers, and landscapers. Her minority preferences extended to her healthcare. Her primary care doctor, Dr. Isaac, was a Black woman whom she had been seeing for years and trusted implicitly. Under Dr. Isaac's guidance, Ms. Engle's hypertension and high cholesterol were well managed, and she was able to keep her weight under reasonable control with a good diet and a regular exercise program.

Over a period of several weeks, Ms. Engle became aware of a growing lump in her groin. She waited until her next appointment with Dr. Isaac, who examined her carefully and diagnosed an inguinal hernia, that is, a weakness in the inguinal canal allowing abdominal contents to protrude. These hernias are not as common in women as in men, and fortunately they are frequently small and don't require an intervention. Nevertheless, Dr. Isaac was concerned by the size of the hernia and the pain it was causing. Ms. Engle was not enthusiastic about having any medical procedures, so they agreed on a period of careful observation, with instructions for Mrs. Engle to call if the lump grew bigger or became even more painful.

Which, unfortunately, it did over the next few weeks. The lump grew to twice the size it had been, and Ms. Engle was having trouble walking without significant pain. Ms. Engle went back to Dr. Isaac, who was unhappy with the progression and advised prompt consultation with a general surgeon. That's when the drama began.

Unsurprisingly, Ms. Engle asked Dr. Isaac to refer her to an African American general surgeon. Dr. Isaac told her that the few she had known and referred patients to had retired. She promised to look into it and call Ms. Engle with a name or two. When Dr. Isaac called Ms. Engle, she sounded frustrated. The two Black surgeons who had practiced in the area and had retired were replaced by Asian physicians. She had no other recommendations.

Ms. Engle was disappointed and promised to search on her own, which turned up no Black surgeons. Her only options were to consult with a non-Black doctor in the area or travel to a Black doctor further away.

After considerable thought, Ms. Engle decided not to betray her longtime preference in care providers and to seek an appointment with a Black general surgeon in a larger town, about an hour's drive away. The first appointment she could secure was three weeks hence. She didn't want to bother Dr. Isaac with more questions or favors and assumed that waiting a few extra days to see the surgeon would not be a problem.

But it was during that waiting period that the worst happened. Ms. Engle was awakened in the middle of the night with severe abdominal pain and vomiting. She called a neighbor who, when she saw Ms. Engle in extreme pain and retching continuously, immediately called 911. The emergency crew wasted little time loading Ms. Engle into their ambulance for the short ride to the local emergency room.

The ER physician who saw Ms. Engle, after learning of her hernia history, had no difficulty diagnosing a bowel obstruction with possible strangulation. He immediately summoned the surgeon on call who happened to be white. Ms. Engle had no trouble agreeing to have the surgeon bring her to the operating room urgently for surgery to fix the hernia and relieve her intestinal obstruction. The surgery went well. The rapidity of the treatment guaranteed that Ms. Engle's bowel suffered no permanent damage and that her recovery would be smooth.

Ms. Engle returned to her job two weeks later, vowing to redouble her efforts not only to recruit more African American students, but also to motivate more of those young people to pursue a career in the healthcare professions.

CASE EXPLANATION

As seen in several stories in this book, medicine is an imprecise science, if it is a science at all. So much of what we do in medicine is to apply statistical averages to individual patients with the hope that each case will proceed somewhat like the norm. And the truth is that diseases don't always play by the rules. Variations in the way diseases present, differences in response to therapy, and deviations from expected prognoses are commonplace, and for various reasons. The experienced clinician knows or intuits these variances and factors them into their care of every patient she evaluates. Most importantly, a good doctor admits uncertainty to the patient and then engages in a detailed discussion of treatment options based on the best prognostication possible. Thus, any treatment decision is "shared" along with the consequences, good or bad.

The expected course of some medical conditions is more difficult to anticipate than others. One of them is the natural history of an inguinal hernia, which was Ms. Engle's affliction. In this common condition, a weakness in the muscles and tendons of the groin allows a portion of the bowel to migrate out of the abdominal cavity. The hernia causes pain and an unsightly bulge, but in most cases, it is not a life-threatening problem.

Therefore, knowing when to intervene to fix a hernia is difficult business, especially in women, in whom this condition is less common than in men. In most cases, patients are diagnosed before they develop severe symptoms. Depending on age and overall medical condition, some patients choose to wait until they develop intractable pain, or the bulge becomes too much to tolerate. Many hernias don't progress and there is a realistic chance that surgery will never be required.

On the other hand, some patients opt to have an operation earlier in the process to avoid complications, a decision made easier with laparoscopic techniques that render the operation an outpatient procedure with low risk and less disability, with a relatively short recovery time.

Fortunately, few patients suffer Ms. Engle's complication. When the bowel becomes entrapped in a weakness in the groin muscles and is squeezed by the surrounding tissue, the bowel becomes obstructed. When it does, it is a true medical emergency. The entrapped bowel will have a compromised circulation and if not freed up within hours, may become "ischemic," meaning the bowel dies from lack of blood flow. In a gangrenous bowel, the barrier between intestinal contents and the blood is breached, allowing bacteria to leak into the circulation, causing life-threatening sepsis.

There was little delay in Mrs. Engle's case. She had been warned by Dr. Isaac to rapidly respond to symptoms that could be compatible with bowel obstruction such as pain and vomiting, and 911 was called quickly. She lived in an area where ambulance response times were short. The ER doctor was also on his toes, made the diagnosis quickly and summoned surgical assistance. Thus, the story ended well. Mrs. Engle's bowel was spared and though she needed an open procedure to relieve the obstruction rather than endoscopy, her recovery was uncomplicated.

When she was first diagnosed with a hernia, Mrs. Engle had been instructed by her primary care doctor to consult with a general surgeon. That didn't necessarily mean she would have had her operation before her bowel obstruction occurred. Unless the surgical consultant detected something in Ms. Engle's presentation that suggested a more imminent problem, it is likely that she would have made the same recommendation of watchful waiting. On the other hand, if the surgeon was worried about bowel entrapment, she might have operated soon. Such a decision might have avoided a bowel obstruction. No operation is entirely safe, but Ms. Engle's subsequent course certainly may have been less traumatic. Regardless, Ms. Engle never made it to the Black surgeon.

Ms. Engle wanted to see a Black surgeon and her insistence on doing so was consistent with her lifetime choices, but it almost cost her her life. She felt much more comfortable with a person who looked like her, and her feelings were not unfounded. There have been several excellent clinical studies in which outcomes are better when patients recognize their caregiver as being like themselves and can place their complete trust in that individual. This pertains not only to race but also to gender and religious background. Unfortunately, Ms. Engle's town was not as racially diverse as many other communities, so finding an African American in any medical specialty was particularly challenging.

COMMENTARY

In our highly developed country, it is hard to believe that getting an appointment to see a doctor can be so difficult. A waiting time of months is not uncommon, especially for the medical subspecialties in which there is a shocking undersupply of doctors. This covers several disciplines, including cardiology, and almost all the surgical sub-specialties. Shortages of neurologists, rheumatologists, and endocrinologists are particularly severe. Savvy medical students avoid these specialties because they don't feature procedures that are likely to generate revenue. Training slots in those disciplines are rarely filled by American medical school graduates.

As we have seen elsewhere in this book, the critical shortage of primary care doctors is the biggest problem of all, with the shortage of general pediatricians not far behind. This has led to a proliferation and even the substitution of physician extenders who are helpful, but only when properly supervised. We have seen the consequences of poorly supervised, functionally independent healthcare providers in another story.

Ms. Engle wanted to consult with an African American surgeon for all the good reasons described earlier. What she and Dr. Isaac discovered is that in many parts of the country, especially theirs, it is nearly impossible to find minority physicians in any specialty. This is particularly the case in surgery and has been for many years. African American heart surgeons, for example, are rare as hen's teeth.

The fact that few African Americans attend and complete medical school and residency training has been recognized for years. Despite enacting policies to attract and enroll minorities, medical schools have made little progress. In the face of drastic shortages of minority professionals, legislators and the judiciary have chosen to hogtie university affirmative action programs. As a direct result, fewer Blacks will gain admission to high quality colleges, the springboard to medical school.

At the same time, it has become abundantly clear that the quality of care of racial minorities in the US is flat-out awful. No matter which metric is used, Blacks are disadvantaged. It is an ugly blight for which no one takes full responsibility. African Americans have a lower life expectancy and a higher mortality from nearly every common and treatable disease. This is because they receive less testing and medical treatment for common diseases in the early stages, allowing disease processes to escalate needlessly to life-threatening proportions. Blacks are less likely to have surgery or procedures to treat diseases, let alone gain access to testing for disease prevention. When their hearts fail, they receive less guideline directed therapy and fewer devices to prevent sudden death. The number of screening colonoscopies in the African American community is a fraction of that observed in whites, though colorectal cancer kills them just as often as it does other racial groups. You can basically forget about preventative dental and eye care for most of the Black population. Their insurance plans don't typically cover dentist and ophthalmologist appointments, and they lack the disposable income to pay for much of it themselves.

African Americans are also grossly under-represented in clinical trials. There are many reasons for this absurd situation, including their understandable wariness about the medical establishment after several well-publicized examples of exploitation of minorities by unscrupulous investigators. In any event, there are several causes for concern over the poor representation of minorities in clinical trials, well beyond the obvious ethical incorrectness. Treatments that may not work as well for minorities are approved and prescribed without hard evidence of benefit and safety. There is a myriad of reasons to believe that racial minorities differ from their white counterparts in disease manifestations and responses to treatment. Extrapolating clinical trial results from studies carried out in a predominantly white population is a disservice to minorities and to the people who care for them. Only recently have regulators put teeth in their requirement to have broad racial representation in trials that are carried out to support a drug or device approval in the United States.

The reaction of the medical establishment to this scandal has been to develop what have been referred to as diversity, respect, equity and inclusion (DREI) programs. Large departments exist in every medical establishment to try to correct the gross imbalance in care that minorities receive. The vice-presidents and associate deans who run these programs collect enormous salaries while overseeing a bloated staff that doesn't even know what its mission is. They mainly "preach to the choir," reminding their veteran medical staff to treat all patients with dignity and respect, as if they ever thought of doing otherwise.

What precisely have these programs accomplished? They will say they have changed the attitude of healthcare workers regarding minorities, and perhaps they have to some small extent. But, for all their efforts and money spent, the disparity in care that I described above is no better and probably even worse than it was before these programs were established. Most importantly, we have seen no increase, and in some cases a decrease, in the number of Blacks who work in the medical professions at any level. The number of Black medical graduates has not increased in proportion to the growth in the African American population, but rather has fallen.

The obvious solution to problems of disparities in care is not to try to change the minds of people who work in hospitals and doctor offices. While there will be bigots in any profession, most healthcare providers are kind, sympathetic, caring people who really don't care about the skin color of their patients. DREI programs that attempt to teach tolerance of minorities may be important in colleges and universities and perhaps in industry and government, but for the medical professions, they are superfluous.

No, the answer to the conundrum of unequal care is to change the constituency of the profession itself. We need orders of magnitude more Black doctors and nurses in our hospitals and offices. The money that is currently being spent on touchy-feely seminars in all-white hospitals needs to be channeled directly into our inner-city elementary and high school systems, to improve the education of Black children at every level. Furthermore, these children need role models. They need to be inspired by successful Black professionals, so they want to become doctors and nurses. Most importantly, they need better facilities and more teachers so they can successfully compete for the higher education they need to achieve their post-graduate goals.

I would submit that Mrs. Engle was prescient. She believed that her medical care and outcomes would be tied not just to the quality of her care but also to her faith and trust in her caregiver. She was convinced that she would do better if she were treated by someone she trusted. We have taken this principle seriously in women's health, but it hasn't yet taken root regarding minorities.

It will take time and reallocation of resources, but we must stop oversimplifying the problem and pretending we have the solution. Platitudes on billboards describing how caring hospital systems are simply won't suffice. It is time to effect real change and that means doing everything we can to increase the number of healthcare providers in poor neighborhoods and motivate minority children to seek out a career in the medical field. We need soldiers to go into the field and care for the people who trust them and need them the most. Abrupt dismantling of diversity programs by the current administration is an obvious mistake. Instead, we need to repurpose these programs to more aggressively foster the development of minority medical students and trainees, to optimize their chance of success, and to encourage them to practice in communities that are in dire need.

CONCLUSION

The medical care of racial minorities in the United States is a disgrace. Everyone knows it. Fixing the situation is not going to be easy and will certainly require a massive reallocation of resources. Healthcare institutions must stop spending money on band-aids like media advertising and self-serving seminars and start establishing primary care clinics in underserved neighborhoods. Medical insurance needs to be affordable and available to everyone, and coverage must include prevention and early disease management. Medical research must broaden its focus to consider how diseases affect minorities and how best to understand that diversity. At the same time, our educational system must be revamped to make higher education, especially medical and nursing school, a realistic goal for all children and to do everything we can to increase the supply of minority practitioners.

PATIENT ADVICE

Only with an increase in the number of minority healthcare providers will we see the development of a wholly improved system of care for all of us, regardless of skin color. And then perhaps Ms. Engle's search for a surgeon who looks like her will no longer be in vain. In the meantime, everyone who wants to see change needs to challenge diversity program advocates to stop wasting resources, to roll up their sleeves to find creative ways to improve healthcare for minorities. DREI programs should not be dismantled as proposed by the current administration. They should be developed and supported so that they focus on what is important and will make a difference in outcomes. So far, they have fallen short. The longer we wait to implement change and continue to politicize the issues, the more likely we will squander the talent and enthusiasm of young people who are eager to move ahead and become the caregivers of the future. Their minds would be a terrible thing to waste.

Story 18: Those Big Centers Love to Tell You Just How Great They Are

"Doctors collectively have done more to block adequate medical care for people in this country than any other single group." —Jimmy Carter

NARRATIVE

Mrs. Lynch was a 48-year-old Caucasian woman and a hard-driving executive type who worked for a large TV/internet company. She was married to a successful corporate lawyer, and the two were quite the power couple. They worked hard and played hard, agreeing at the beginning of their courtship not to have children so they could maximize the things they enjoyed the most, like traveling extensively and eating out at premier restaurants. They circulated in the best social circles and were frequently invited to parties given by the most important people. They both enjoyed sports, playing as well as watching. In addition to membership at an elite gym, they could be seen sitting in the front row of basketball games or right behind home plate when their hometown baseball team was in the playoffs. By all accounts, they were living the good life. Mrs. Lynch's one notable flaw was a tendency to over-worry and obsess, a neurosis she worked hard her entire life to overcome, mostly unsuccessfully.

One afternoon, while at a business conference in Chicago, Mrs. Lynch had the sudden onset of palpitations. She felt rapid and irregular heart action along with just a bit of lightheadedness and a feeling of dread. She excused herself from the conference and made for the restroom, but the palpitations stopped before she got there, and she immediately felt better. She was able to finish the meeting and her trip, albeit with sweaty palms during the flight back home.

Though worried about what had happened, Mrs. Lynch decided to wait to see if the episode recurred before seeing her doctor. It turned out that she had no further symptoms, and after several weeks, she had all but forgotten about the Chicago event. When she finally saw her internist, Dr. Keats, a few weeks later, she mentioned it only in passing. Dr. Keats was concerned by her description of the symptoms, fearing that she might have had atrial fibrillation, an important cardiac arrhythmia that could cause a stroke. She ordered a few tests, including a measure of her thyroid function and an echocardiogram, both of which were normal. She also recommended a Holter monitor, a device that Mrs. Lynch would wear for twenty-four hours to determine if her rhythm was normal, and it was. At her follow-up visit, Mrs. Lynch and Dr. Keats decided to hold off on a cardiac referral or further work-up at least for the time being.

A few nights later, while watching the evening news with her husband, Mrs. Lynch saw a TV commercial advertising a relatively inexpensive device she could use to record her heart rhythm. The device could be ordered online with a home delivery the next day, and, according to the announcer, it was approved by the FDA for detecting atrial fibrillation, a potentially fatal arrhythmia. The "doctor" in the white coat said it was easy to use, requiring only brief index finger contact to generate a high-quality tracing that could be transmitted to a doctor's office and stored on a cell phone. He encouraged the viewer to get the device and use it before it was "too late."

Mrs. Lynch called Dr. Keats's office and asked her nurse if purchasing the device was a good idea. The answer was an unqualified yes; there would be little harm in having the gadget available. In fact, the nurse recommended that Mrs. Lynch make a habit of recording her heart rhythm a few times a day, even if she wasn't having symptoms, just to make sure all was well.

Mrs. Lynch did exactly what the nurse suggested. She bought the device, familiarized herself with how to use it, and began to record her heart rhythm many times a day, from the time she rose in the morning to bedtime at night, even waking up to make sure her heart rhythm was normal. After several days of this obsession, she finally found something. During a recording in the early afternoon at her office, while she felt perfectly well, the device indicated that her heart was out of rhythm. The episode lasted for fifteen seconds, and her heart rate during that time was recorded on the device as 160 beats per minute.

Mrs. Lynch called Dr. Keats' office and transmitted the recording for her review. Dr. Keats returned the call after reviewing the strip and recommended that Mrs. Lynch schedule an appointment with a cardiac electrophysiologist, also known as a heart rhythm specialist. The rhythm she had recorded was indeed atrial fibrillation. She would need to immediately start taking an anticoagulant, a blood thinner, to prevent a stroke, and a beta blocker to keep her heart rate under control. Dr. Keats would send the prescriptions to Mrs. Lynch's pharmacy.

Dr. Keats also told her she would almost certainly need an ablation procedure. Dr. Keats briefly explained that this was a catheter procedure during which the specialist would identify and cauterize the area from which the arrhythmia originated. There were several places locally that did many of these procedures, and Dr. Keats suggested a specialist to whom she had referred several patients. Those she had sent to him had done well and were pleased with his bedside skills and compassion. Dr. Keats emphasized that she favored this electrophysiologist because he was conservative and only recommended procedures when they were necessary and there were no other reasonable alternatives. He would also talk to her about the need to continue taking blood thinners and other medications. If Mrs. Lynch wanted to see him, Dr. Keats would be happy to make the referral.

Mrs. Lynch didn't receive the news well at all. In fact, the idea that she might need an ablation procedure and was at risk of having a stroke threw her into a panic. Immediately after hanging up with Dr. Keats, she began a frantic search of the internet, looking for information about atrial fibrillation and ablation. There was much to peruse. Not only was atrial fibrillation a common arrhythmia, but experts at all the prestigious centers in the United States touted cardiac ablation as the preferred method of treatment. Some, like a famous clinic in the Midwest, boasted that their rates of success were higher and their complication rates lower than anywhere else in the world, one of the leading reasons why their cardiac center was ranked number one in the US. Furthermore, this center was pioneering several new methods of performing ablations that would "revolutionize" the technique and make it even more effective, safe and fast. Consultation with one of their electrophysiologists was easy to arrange with a single phone call or email.

Mrs. Lynch spent the rest of the day on her atrial fibrillation research and was loaded with information when her husband arrived home. She briefed him over dinner, answering his many questions as best she could from the information she had garnered from online sources. She explained why she was so worried about her diagnosis. Stroke and heart failure are frequent events in AF patients, and she wanted nothing to do with either of those terrible diagnoses.

When the dishes were done and they finally relaxed in their sitting room, Mr. Lynch offered to call his brother, an orthopedic surgeon in Pittsburgh, to gather advice and insight from someone inside the profession.

Brother Jim was happy to hear Mr. Lynch's voice. They had been close as children, but both now had busy lives that limited contact to holidays and special occasions. After a few minutes of small talk, Mr. Lynch asked Jim if he knew anything about atrial fibrillation and catheter ablation. Jim admitted he didn't know much, but from what he had heard, it was a rapidly evolving technique. He recommended trying to find a place that had cutting-edge technology in addition to vast experience, to maximize the chances of a good outcome. Jim also told Mr. Lynch that getting an ablation was a very good idea since it offered the best chance of "curing" the arrhythmia. When Mr. Lynch mentioned the midwestern center as a possible site for the procedure, Brother Jim heartily endorsed the idea. He knew several people who had traveled from Pittsburgh to have heart procedures there, and as far as he knew, they were happy with the outcomes.

Jim's opinion immediately resonated with Mrs. Lynch. It jibed well with what she had learned during her internet search. After notifying Dr. Keats of their decision to travel west, Mr. and Mrs. Lynch booked an appointment for the following week with the co-director of the cardiac ablation laboratory.

Armed with a long list of questions and concerns, Mr. and Mrs. Lynch arrived early for their appointment and were offered a beverage while they waited for the doctor in a consultation room. They were immediately impressed with the well-spoken and well-kempt Dr. Wolf who, after a brief review of her history and a cursory physical examination, began a lengthy discourse about her disease and all the options for treatment.

Dr. Wolf reinforced the need to suppress atrial fibrillation to avoid its dreaded complications, particularly a stroke that, at Mrs. Lynch's age, would be catastrophic. He affirmed the preeminence of catheter ablation as a first line treatment. He stated emphatically that he did not recommend antiarrhythmic drugs as initial treatment for Mrs. Lynch. Given her age and relatively good health, in his opinion it would be best to "eradicate" the arrhythmia by destroying the cells that were generating it. He echoed her brother-in-law Jim's reassurance that a cure was achievable. If complete arrhythmia suppression could be achieved, Dr. Wolf said she wouldn't need to be on anticoagulants for the rest of her life and likely wouldn't need to take any medications. Mrs. Lynch was pleased to hear the news, particularly because the beta blocker that had been prescribed was causing unusual fatigue and listlessness.

The next question from Mrs. Lynch was where the ablation would best be carried out. She was aware of The Clinic's prowess, but she was concerned about the logistics of traveling for the procedure. Dr. Wolf was ready with his reply, reassuring Mrs. Lynch that his center was her best choice and that, over the years, his department had perfected the logistics of having cardiac procedures. A hotel for the couple's use before and after the procedure was right next to the hospital, and he anticipated a stay of only a couple days before she returned home arrhythmia-free. Back home, her local cardiologist would see to her follow-up care, but Dr. Wolf reassured the couple that he would be available to them and her doctors for any questions or issues.

Dr. Wolf then went on to explain the procedure in detail, including the use of a new energy source called pulsed field ablation (PFA). He said that The Clinic had pioneered this newly approved method to destroy the cardiac tissue responsible for the arrhythmia. Instead of burning or freezing, PFA lysed cells by destroying their membranes. This would result in less damage to contiguous structures, better efficacy, and shorter procedure time. Dr. Wolf emphasized that no center in the world had more experience with PFA than his, and their results were "stellar."

Their consultation completed, Mr. and Mrs. Lynch headed for the airport. By the time they boarded their flight, they had decided that they would return there for the procedure as soon as it could be scheduled. Three weeks later, Mrs. Lynch was on a gurney, lightly sedated, and headed into the electrophysiology laboratory, chock full of state-of-the-art technology, to rid her of her dangerous arrhythmia.

As Dr. Wolf had predicted, the procedure was carried off flawlessly. In a little less than three hours, catheters had been withdrawn from Mrs. Lynch's veins, and she was in the recovery unit, husband at her side, regaining full consciousness. Dr. Wolf arrived in good spirits, announcing that her arrhythmia had been effectively dealt with. Given what he had seen in the laboratory, he was convinced that it would not recur and all would be well.

The flight home two days later was a joyous occasion for Mr. and Mrs. Lynch. They congratulated themselves for so carefully navigating their way through the arrhythmia problem and finding a definitive solution. Given the whirlwind of the previous two days, for their first night at home they decided to order Chinese take-out, watch a movie and retire early.

However, in the wee hours of the morning, Mrs. Lynch awoke with excruciating chest tightness and pain radiating into her jaw. She broke into a cold sweat and vomited her dinner on their bedroom carpet. Mr. Lynch immediately called 911. The paramedics took a brief history and then did an electrocardiogram, which they said showed "abnormal findings." They started an IV, administered nitroglycerin, which provided some relief, and loaded Mrs. Lynch into an ambulance. The trip to the local hospital was short, and the interventional cardiology fellow on call was already in the ER when Mrs. Lynch was wheeled in, anxious to know if emergency cardiac catheterization would be necessary for a suspected heart attack.

The fellow told Mrs. Lynch, and her husband, who had driven over separately, that she might indeed be having a heart attack, but the electrocardiogram was not typical of a major vessel blockage. He told the couple he had presented the case to his attending physician, who was off site, and had transmitted her electrocardiogram to him. The senior doctor said he preferred to wait for her cardiac enzyme levels before deciding if she needed a catheterization. The values would indicate if she was having a heart attack. When the couple reminded the fellow that Mrs. Lynch had just returned home after having an AF ablation in another city, he said he didn't see anything that indicated a procedural complication, but he would perform an echocardiogram to make sure she didn't have fluid around the outside of her heart or damage to her heart valves caused by the procedure.

Ms. Lynch was taken to an observation area. Although the echocardiogram was a technically difficult study, the fellow didn't see evidence that the ablation catheters had poked a hole in her heart causing blood to leak into the heart's lining, and her heart valves were intact. But when the cardiac enzyme levels came back distinctly elevated, the fellow informed the attending physician, who told him to call in the catheterization laboratory team while he dressed and drove to the hospital. They would need to perform a catheter test to exclude a coronary artery occlusion. As an aside, he also told the fellow to ask the patient what energy source had been used for the ablation procedure.

While the laboratory was being set up, the attending physician conferred with the cardiology fellow and learned that Mrs. Lynch's procedure had used PFA. He then came to Mrs. Lynch's bedside, and after introducing himself and reassuring the couple, he explained to them that an unusual but recognized complication of pulsed field ablation was spasm of one of the coronary arteries, usually the vessel that supplied the lateral surface of the heart. No one understood completely why this happened and it was hard to know how often it occurred because the technique was so new. However, the time course was consistent, as were the enzyme elevations and subtle electrocardiogram findings.

If coronary artery spasm was the cause here, it would be necessary to place a catheter into the artery and attempt to open it up with medication or possibly with a stent. In the meantime, he ordered a drip of nitroglycerin, which he hoped would reduce the coronary spasm at least enough to preserve heart muscle until catheters were in place to deliver medications directly into the blocked artery.

In very little time, less than an hour, Mrs. Lynch was on the catheterization table with a coronary catheter in place showing that the circumflex coronary artery that supplied the left side of the heart was almost completely closed off. The pattern of occlusion and its location in the circumflex artery suggested that the cause was spasm of the artery and not an atherosclerotic plaque. Indeed, when nitroglycerin and other vasodilating drugs were administered directly into the vessel, it slowly opened, Mrs. Lynch's chest discomfort fully abated and her electrocardiogram returned to normal.

Bloodwork and other tests subsequently carried out indicated that Mrs. Lynch had suffered a moderate amount of heart damage from the coronary occlusion, but much less than if the problem had not been dealt with expeditiously. The cardiologist who had wisely intervened admitted to the couple that there had been a delay in activating the catheterization laboratory team because her ECG abnormality was subtle. Suspicion of coronary disease had been low since she was young with no real risk factors for coronary artery disease and the fellow on call was unaware of the potential for coronary artery spasm with PFA.

He explained that the circumflex artery supplied blood to the side of the heart that wasn't as easily seen during the electrocardiogram or echocardiogram recording. It wasn't until the enzyme tests came back and he learned that her ablation energy source was pulsed field that he realized that the circumflex artery might be in spasm. It so happened that the circumflex artery traveled very close to the area where AF ablation energy had been applied. How did he know of that potential complication? His colleagues who carried out ablations at his hospital had decided not to employ ultra-new technology like PFA until the kinks were worked out, one of which was this serious problem of circumflex coronary artery spasm.

Mrs. Lynch made a good recovery and was just about ready for discharge when, to her chagrin, she had a three-minute episode of AF on the monitor associated with mild symptoms of palpitations and breathlessness. The cardiologist understood how disappointed she was to have a recurrence after all she had gone through. He explained that AF in the few weeks after an ablation is not uncommon and doesn't necessarily mean that the procedure failed. Also, the arrhythmia may have been triggered by cardiac irritability associated with her heart attack. There was no way to know what the future would hold in this regard, but he promised to take very good care of his new patient. Above all, Mrs. Lynch and he agreed that this time around, no matter what, conservative management closer to her home would be the order of the day.

CASE EXPLANATION

Mrs. Lynch had AF, of that there was no doubt. The major question in her case was how best to manage it. Remember that she had had only a couple of episodes, and her symptoms were not severe. In fact, the arrhythmia was first recorded when she was asymptomatic. Given her age, good general health, and lack of cardiac risk factors such as diabetes, hypertension, or heart failure, her risk of stroke or heart failure was low, so a period of watchful waiting would have been totally appropriate along with a large dose of reassurance. Her symptoms might have increased over time, but the natural history of AF is highly variable. Patients can have long inter-episode intervals and not require any intervention for months or years. When her family doctor told the worry-prone Mrs. Lynch about stroke and heart failure, she greatly exacerbated her anxiety, causing her unnecessary distress.

In the early phases of AF, if patients have symptoms severe enough to warrant treatment, antiarrhythmic drugs are useful. They work well and provide an observation time, during which the patient can get used to the idea of having a chronic disease. Many patients can use antiarrhythmic drugs periodically, at the time of a recurrence, to shorten the time they have the arrhythmia and to relieve their symptoms. Various antiarrhythmic drug options would have been available for Mrs. Lynch. Though they were mentioned by Dr. Wolf during her initial consultation, he opined that none of them were as appropriate as a catheter ablation procedure.

Mrs. Lynch also did not need an anticoagulant drug. By virtue of being young and healthy, she was at low risk of a stroke, so any argument that ridding her of the arrhythmia with an ablation procedure would help her avoid the complications of blood thinners was inappropriate. Likewise, Dr. Keats, who first prescribed the anticoagulant, exposed her to the risk of a major bleeding event for no gain. Furthermore, Mrs. Lynch's risk of heart failure with infrequent and short AF episodes was very low, especially if her heart rate was well controlled.

As so often happens in medicine, Mrs. Lynch was grossly overtreated not only with the blood thinner but also with the beta blocker that did little except make her tired and irritable. Her primary care doctor, even though she introduced the idea of an early ablation procedure prematurely, did make the correct diagnosis and recommended consultation with someone she trusted to be fair and conservative. Mrs. Lynch, with an abundance of misinformation from the internet, and off-the-cuff advice from her uninformed brother-in-law, went elsewhere to pursue the idea of a "cure." The electrophysiologist there was only too happy to schedule a procedure without a balanced discussion of her alternatives. Not only was the young doctor eager for cases to increase his clinical volume, but he was anxious to use his new toy, pulsed field ablation, on patients so he could publish his results and become famous. The healthy and naïve Mrs. Lynch, with a normal heart, a short history of AF, and unrealistic expectations, was perfect for his purposes. In his enthusiasm, he failed to inform Mr. and Mrs. Lynch that PFA ablation was as fraught with the same risks of early recurrence as more standard techniques, or that PFA ablation had unique risks including coronary artery vasospasm.

As we saw, Mrs. Lynch developed vasospasm of one of the three main coronary arteries. Given the relative newness of the technique, it is difficult to know exactly how often this dreaded complication will occur and why.

We also don't know how to predict which patients are more likely to have it, and, of course, how to prevent it. Only a few months after approval of PFA ablation devices, one company's machines were recalled by the FDA after an unexpectedly high number of serious adverse events, once again illustrating the wisdom of letting other doctors use new technology before adopting it. More recently, a randomized trial documented more serious adverse events with PFA than with conventional radiofrequency ablation, with no evidence of added benefit. Sir William Osler's admonition to use new therapies while they still worked would apply perfectly to Mrs. Lynch's case.

The cardiology fellow who saw Mrs. Lynch when she had her heart attack was not familiar with coronary artery spasm as a complication of PFA ablation. This fact, plus the atypical electrocardiogram, delayed the intervention that eventually opened the coronary artery that had gone into spasm. Fortunately, Mrs. Lynch didn't suffer a large amount of heart damage from her vessel closure. Her heart function on subsequent echocardiograms appeared nearly normal and she was asymptomatic from that perspective. How a scar in her heart will impact her cardiac status and prognosis over the course of time is not knowable.

Did the PFA ablation work for Mrs. Lynch? Sadly, it didn't. Not only did she have an early recurrence, but she went on to have monthly episodes of palpitations lasting from a few minutes to an hour with symptoms of palpitations and some breathlessness. She was able to function during the arrhythmias, but she didn't like the way she felt. Her new cardiologist eventually placed her on an old and highly effective generic drug called dofetilide, which reduced the AF frequency enough to satisfy Mrs. Lynch. She tolerated the drug well and continued to take it chronically. Her cardiologist was pleased with the response but when Mrs. Lynch asked him why this or any antiarrhythmic drug wasn't recommended before the ablation procedure, he would only smile, shrug his shoulders and say he didn't know. Or maybe he did, and like many doctors, didn't want to impugn the reputation of a colleague.

COMMENTARY

Every year, *U.S. News & World Report* publishes lists of what they have judged to be the best hospitals in the country overall, and by subspecialty. It also ranks hospitals regionally using similar metrics. Exactly how a hospital or medical center wins a spot in the top fifty is difficult to know for sure, but the most important metric appears to be reputation. The more widely known the medical center, the more likely they will place in the upper tier and stay there for years.

Medical institutions establish their reputation mainly by publishing in high profile scientific journals. Doing that requires cutting-edge research, usually funded by industry or the government. These research efforts are expensive. Large grants allow institutions to hire armies of researchers and technicians and house them in well-equipped facilities with the expectation that they will discover new ways to diagnose and treat disease. When these "breakthroughs" are published in prestigious journals and presented at international meetings, people take notice. That includes people in the media who love to tell the public how a new study result will change the course of medical treatment and save countless lives. If only a fraction of these medical advances worked as well as touted, humans would likely be immortal.

Despite the hype, healthcare providers and patients alike assume, correctly in some cases, that the institutions mentioned repeatedly in the press deliver the best and most effective care for patients and are worthy of the legion of referrals and consultations that their reputations elicit. Unquestionably, these centers should be available for patients who have relatively rare or difficult diseases given their experience and access to the latest technology.

Before social media and the proliferation of medical coverage by the lay press, reputational referral was an insider's game. Doctors called doctors to refer their patients to the places they knew could deliver cutting-edge therapy for rare or complex diseases. Communication was key, because passing a patient back and forth between providers, usually in a remote city or state, can be rife with error. Doctors understood that well and took precautions to make transitions of care as smooth as possible. Essential elements in seamless care used to be the phone call and the learned referral letter, neither of which is still in vogue.

But the healthcare behemoths weren't satisfied with just being a good and reliable referral center for individual practitioners who had sick patients with rare or complex diseases. They wanted more of everything: patients, money, luxurious buildings, and prestige. To get more, they went on the offensive. Instead of waiting for physicians to call them to refer patients, they began to solicit. They found that bragging in the media about all they could do was a productive strategy, and they used it to the maximum, even paying for TV commercial time in markets far from their catchment area.

As a result, patients travelled to these centers on their own, drawn by the promise of better care of what was usually a common disease, and because it was assumed that outcomes would be better at Mecca Medical Center. When carefully evaluated, however, there has been no consistent evidence of superiority. Hard outcomes data have shown no difference in the chances of success or the incidence of complications at top-tier sites compared to other large volume centers. What was clear was that the influx of patients to these centers permitted them to increase their clinical research volume to further enhance their reputation.

Still not satisfied with their success, elite medical centers went even further, selling their name to lesser institutions that wanted to enhance their reputations regionally. Thus, it would now be possible to get MD Anderson Cancer caliber care at a regional hospital without having to travel to Houston. State-of-the-art cardiology treatment would now be available at an otherwise average hospital in the middle of nowhere. Exactly how such wonderful quality would be infused into the smaller and lesser equipped and staffed hospitals was not a part of the TV commercial that touted the idea. Most importantly, there was no need to prove that the quality was better with these casual associations. It was just another example of inflated medical advertising.

But media campaigning has not been limited to large centers. All hospital administrators came to believe that they would also be able to enhance their business by advertising in local media. The early adopters were looked at askance. For decades, doctors believed that advertising services was unethical. Those who dared to place ads were quickly ostracized. But the fear of being left out eventually drove just about every medical center to produce and air commercials. And since commercials were unregulated, content quickly became unplugged with undocumented claims and reckless promises. It was not considered at all inappropriate for a small hospital to declare preeminence in any field it chose. Terms like "cutting edge," "state-of-the-art" and "world class" were so common as to be banal.

The lemming-like stampede to advertising would be humorous if it hadn't caused hundreds of millions to be spent annually on marketing programs that do nothing to improve patient care. Ironically, given the sheer volume of medical advertising, the public has come to ignore just about anything hospitals have to say since their messages are uniformly grandiose. How many people who watched the Super Bowl remember that a prominent medical center advertised its cardiac services during a time out? Exactly what did that medical center expect to get out of bragging to tens of millions of guacamole-and-beer-guzzling football fanatics, and did they really think the enormous price for their thirty seconds of fame was worth it?

Once hospitals opened the floodgates of advertising, it wasn't long before physician groups and even individual practitioners took to the media. Right next to shameless plaintiff malpractice attorney billboards are ads with photos of smiling cardiologists who encourage you to go to their hospital if you are having a heart attack, as if you will have the time to review your many options.

And it seems that there are no limits on medical advertising content. Rogue medical professionals, or actors impersonating doctors or nurses, advertise bogus, unproven or debunked treatments, all with the goal of soliciting paying patients. Testimonials by washed-up celebrities who are happy to relate how their lives were saved or improved by some specious treatments are common and particularly disgraceful. I wonder if those football players on television ever asked the purveyors exactly how a copper band placed around the waist relieves back pain before they advised the public to buy one.

CONCLUSION

The advent of the internet and social media has had a major impact on patient care, as it has on almost every aspect of modern life. Patients have been empowered to make more decisions about their healthcare. Much of this is a positive change. Patients with a better knowledge of their disease and their treatment options would be expected to fare better.

Unfortunately, not all the information that is available to patients is helpful. The internet is peppered with misinformation about common and uncommon medical conditions. Some of that misrepresentation is viciously intentional, with the goal of purveying expensive treatments that provide no real hope of benefit. Contributing to the confusion is naivete and a lack of fundamental knowledge. It is simply impossible for patients to navigate their way through the piles of information that a search engine provides and arrive at a learned decision about their healthcare. Deciding on a treatment option is difficult enough, but the important decision about where to pursue care is just as complicated and frequently contaminated. Profligate advertising not only wastes money but misdirects patients and contributes nothing to the quality of medical care.

PATIENT ADVICE

In this story, an intelligent and highly educated woman decided to go to a distant medical center to have her arrhythmia treated because of its reputation. Unfortunately, she suffered complications, and the fragmentation of her care led to delayed treatment. Seeking help from a distinguished medical center under some circumstances, for example, to treat a rare disease may be a very good idea. But arriving at a good decision requires excellent communication with properly motivated and principled healthcare providers on all sides of the referral process. As we have seen in other stories, whatever can be done to prevent care fragmentation should be the highest priority.

Story # 19: Medical Clearance or How to Blame Somebody Else

"Medicine is the science of uncertainty and the art of probability."
—Sir William Osler

NARRATIVE

Mr. Coyle was a 63-year-old Caucasian businessman who took his healthcare seriously. He had hypertension and diabetes, so he and his internist agreed that he would not only have a quarterly physical examination and laboratory testing, but that he would have his prostate checked regularly, get regular cardiac stress testing, and have colon cancer screening every five years. This was particularly important because Mr. Coyle's father had died of colon cancer and polyps had been discovered during his previous colonoscopies.

Two years later, when he was 65, his primary care doctor detected an irregular heart rhythm and diagnosed atrial fibrillation. Fortunately for Mr. Coyle, he had no symptoms and his heart rate was not excessive, so the only treatment he needed was a blood thinner, which he took faithfully and with no side effects.

When the time came for Mr. Coyle's surveillance colonoscopy, his gastroenterologist, Dr. Wynn, insisted that he be evaluated by a cardiologist, and referred him to Dr. Singh, one of his partners in a multi-specialty group. Dr. Wynn was concerned about Mr. Coyle's high blood pressure and diabetes and wanted to be certain that Mr. Coyle was getting optimal treatment for atrial fibrillation. He was particularly concerned because Mr. Coyle was using an anticoagulant to prevent a stroke. Dr. Wynn wanted "cardiac clearance" for the colonoscopy that would include instructions about management of the anticoagulant before and after the procedure. Dr. Singh's office confirmed that he would be able to see Mr. Coyle and deliver an opinion within a week so as not to delay the colonoscopy procedure.

At his appointment, Dr. Singh spent about ten minutes with Mr. Coyle.

He asked a few perfunctory questions, looked at Mr. Coyle's electrocardiogram and said that Mr. Coyle was going to need some tests before the colonoscopy. He ordered a stress test with nuclear imaging, an echocardiogram and a 24-hour Holter monitor to check his heart rhythm. He told Mr. Coyle that all the studies could be carried out at the group's office in the next few days and, if the results were acceptable, he could then have his colonoscopy.

Mr. Coyle was taken aback. He had no symptoms, and his medical issues were under excellent control. Dr. Singh said he agreed but he needed the tests to make sure everything would go smoothly. Without the tests, he would not be able to "clear" Mr. Coyle for colonoscopy.

Reluctantly, Mr. Coyle had the tests but instead of a few days, it took a month to complete them. When he finally saw the results on a patient portal, he was alarmed. There were several items of concern, but he couldn't make much sense of them. A week later, Dr. Singh's office finally called. An office nurse told him he had continuous atrial fibrillation, but his heart rate was "controlled." He performed well on the stress test, but the nuclear imaging portion was abnormal, showing an area of poor perfusion on the under surface of the heart compatible with a scar. That finding correlated with a wall motion abnormality in the same area on the echocardiogram. The nurse instructed Mr. Coyle to have a CAT scan of his coronary arteries to look for blockages before he could proceed with the colonoscopy. When Mr. Coyle asked about the seriousness of the problem, the nurse told Mr. Coyle that Dr. Singh thought that these findings could represent a major problem. If the CAT scan revealed coronary artery disease, he would likely need open-heart surgery or a stent.

Mr. Coyle and his wife now were very upset. His primary care doctor had told him repeatedly that he was in good health; now he was being told he might have significant disease of his coronary arteries and need a major procedure.

After several more weeks of waiting and worrying, Mr. Coyle had the CAT scan and learned a few days later that the results were negative. His coronary arteries had a few plaques but no significant blockages. He could proceed with the colonoscopy as planned.

Dr. Singh's nurse practitioner, who called him with the CAT scan results, advised Mr. Coyle to stop his blood thinner two days before the colonoscopy and to restart it "as soon as possible" after the procedure. Since he had a history of colon polyps requiring removal, she explained to Mr. Coyle that interrupting the anticoagulant for a short period would reduce the chances of bleeding from the colon after the procedure.

Mr. Coyle stopped his blood thinner for two days before his colonoscopy, which went off as scheduled and without incident. He had two polyps that Dr. Wynn was able to extract. After the procedure, Dr. Wynn told Mr. Coyle that the polyps had been "sessile" or flattened against the wall of the colon and therefore relatively difficult to remove. Consequently, there was some local bleeding in the wall of the colon that took a while to control. Dr. Wynn told Mr. Coyle not to restart his blood thinner for five days to give his gut wall a chance to heal.

Three days after the colonoscopy, Mr. Coyle awoke with numbness in his right arm. When he attempted to get out of bed, he fell because he had no strength in his right leg. He tried to rouse his wife, but he couldn't find the words. He finally got her attention, and when it was clear to both that something was badly wrong, she called 911. Within minutes, he was in his local hospital's emergency room where he was seen by a neurologist. An MRI indicated that he had had an "ischemic stroke," meaning that a clot in a vessel in his brain had caused him to lose function in the part of the brain supplied by that vessel, in his case, the left side of his brain.

Based on his presentation and timing, Mr. Coyle was treated appropriately with a clot buster drug called TPA and placed in the intensive care unit. Over the next several hours, his neurological status stabilized but he remained weak and unable to speak clearly. His wife called his speech a "word salad" because he used familiar words but without proper syntax or meaning.

During his hospitalization, Mrs. Coyle, who was a retired nurse, asked the treating neurologist what had caused the stroke. The neurologist explained that since Mr. Coyle had atrial fibrillation, she believed that a clot had developed in the heart's non-functioning upper chamber, had broken off, and then traveled to the brain occluding a major blood vessel and depriving the brain of blood flow. The clot buster drug probably helped but couldn't restore blood flow fast enough to prevent brain damage, some of which might be permanent.

Mrs. Coyle asked why, if her husband had been susceptible to a blood clot in the brain, had his anticoagulant drug been interrupted and not restarted promptly by Dr. Wynn after the colonoscopy. To her chagrin, the neurologist said she didn't know and declined to speculate. She recommended a conversation with Dr. Wynn.

Mr. Coyle was ultimately discharged to a rehabilitation facility, where he learned to use a walker and recovered some of his speech. Despite excellent care, he didn't return to normal function. He lost his job and was permanently disabled, having to depend on his wife and family for custodial care.

Mrs. Coyle did eventually speak with all the doctors about what had happened to her husband. She didn't believe she was getting precise or honest answers. The situation came to a head when Dr. Singh and Dr. Wynn stopped returning her calls. Reluctantly, on the advice of a close friend and neighbor, she decided to consult a personal injury law firm.

CASE EXPLANATION

Mr. Coyle suffered a disabling stroke, a catastrophic event that for most patients is scarier than dying. The stroke occurred because the blood thinning drug he had been using chronically and successfully to prevent a blood clot from leaving his dysfunctional left atrium and going to the brain was interrupted so he could have a colonoscopy. The gastroenterologist sent Mr. Coyle to a cardiologist in his own group. He did so as a matter of course. All patients who had any kind of cardiac risk were referred for what was called "clearance," but what was really supposed to be an evaluation of cardiovascular risk.

Pre-operative and pre-procedure screening is ubiquitous in the community, being used before nearly any invasive medical or surgical procedure including cataract extraction, dermatological procedures and many others for which the surgical risk is minimal. Billions of dollars are spent on what is commonly called "cardiac clearance." Unfortunately, there is no evidence that cardiac testing or treatment of stable patients before any procedure, including joint replacement or major abdominal or chest surgery, prevents clinical events such as heart attacks, strokes or cardiovascular death. The axiom in professional society guidelines is that if the patient is stable, without any recent cardiovascular events, most procedures can be carried out with minimal risk, and that pre-operative testing or a radical change in treatment is not helpful.

The evaluation by the cardiologist in this case was not only unnecessary but, predictably, led to several other tests that Mr. Coyle didn't need. As frequently happens, muddy results led to further expensive testing that in the end yielded nothing of consequence. Focused on turning the revenue crank, Dr. Singh failed to personally address the most important issue for Mr. Coyle, blood thinner management. Instead, it was left to the nurse practitioner to instruct Mr. Coyle. She didn't adequately explain why the drug had to be interrupted. More importantly, she never told Mr. Coyle about the unavoidable risk of doing so. Compounding the error, Dr. Singh didn't tell Dr. Wynn to call if there was any reason to withhold the anticoagulant longer than a few hours after the procedure, as is usual.

Dr. Wynn erred by not informing Dr. Singh about his decision to delay resuming the blood thinner because of colon bleeding, even though they were in the same practice. Despite performing colonoscopies on scores of patients with atrial fibrillation, Dr. Wynn didn't understand how dangerous any interruption of anticoagulation can be and so didn't explain his decision to Mr. Coyle and his wife. In essence, Dr. Singh and Dr. Wynn relied on a flawed referral paradigm that failed to account for a patient whose most important clinical problem, susceptibility to stroke, was never adequately addressed by the doctors or with the patient.

The personal injury law firm had no difficulty sorting things out. They faulted the cardiologist, Dr. Singh, for not explaining the problem of anticoagulant interruption to Mr. Coyle and for not providing precise instructions to the gastroenterologist, Dr. Wynn. They blamed Dr. Wynn for blithely recommending a longer period of drug interruption than usual without speaking with the cardiologist. Even worse, none of the anticoagulation instructions given to Mr. Coyle were recorded in his chart by anyone.

What the lawyers didn't understand or chose not to process was that interruption of anticoagulation is a common event in clinical practice and that the risk of stroke over a few days is very low, much less than one percent. Furthermore, there is no easy remedy. To avoid morbid bleeding, blood thinners must be withdrawn for at least two days before surgeries and procedures. Therefore, informing the patient about the finite and irreducible hazard of interrupting the anticoagulant is vitally important. Full disclosure allows the patient to choose between cancelling the procedure or taking the very small risk of having a stroke. This is particularly important for elective procedures like plastic surgery, in which the benefit may not be enough to outweigh a mortal risk. A colonoscopy was a good idea for Mr. Coyle, given his family and personal gastrointestinal history. His consent to proceed likely would not have been altered by an appropriately full disclosure of risk.

The lawsuit dragged on in the courts for five years. It was kept alive mainly because Mr. and Mrs. Coyle were infuriated by the shameless practice of referring patients to partners for money-generating consultations and unnecessary tests, leaving out the most important elements of care. The plaintiffs also profited from finger pointing, as the cardiologist and gastroenterologist blamed each other for the adverse outcome. Dr. Wynn insisted that Dr. Singh should have explained the situation to the patient, while Dr. Singh insisted that his nurse practitioner did her job by telling the patient to restart the anticoagulant "as soon as possible." Discovery and depositions continued with endless experts contributing highly charged opinions that encouraged all attorneys involved to dig in and bill for more hours rather than negotiating a settlement.

After years of posturing, the case was settled for a few million dollars, 40 percent of which went to the plaintiff's attorneys. At least some of the money would be used to provide necessary care for a disabled man for several years. None of the principals in the case were made to admit guilt, but each knew that they would face increased malpractice premiums in addition to adverse publicity. They were also enlightened. The way they would treat patients presenting with similar issues in the future would be forever changed.

COMMENTARY

As we have seen several times in this book, medical care in the United States is absurdly expensive and the quality is not commensurate with the cost. Of the several reasons for this, perhaps the vilest is intentional fraud, as often occurs in disability claims. Obviously, when people are injured on the job, they deserve compensation. The problem is that a large percentage of claims are either entirely false or greatly exaggerated. Since the cost of supporting an injured individual for years is extraordinary, a system has been developed to have claimants thoroughly evaluated and examined before benefits are approved. We now have a vast network of companies and healthcare professionals whose entire job is to process claims and carry out tests to weed out those unsupported claims. In essence, the system spends hundreds of millions of dollars to inspect claims to save billions of dollars that would have been paid to cheaters.

As sad as disability abuse is, by sheer volume needless referral and testing are even higher on the list of wasteful practices. There are several reasons for this ubiquitous practice pattern. Most relevant is the fear of being sued for a bad outcome. Surgeons and proceduralists like Dr. Wynn hold the misguided belief that if they can get another physician to "clear" a patient for a procedure, they will be less culpable for a poor outcome. Shifting blame is a poor strategy in a malpractice lawsuit. Finger-pointing, as it is referred to in the legal community, is a plaintiff malpractice lawyer's fondest dream because it virtually ensures a payout, no matter how weak the case.

Even more absurd is the expansion in the reasons for cardiac consultation. Originally, cardiac screening was for patients about to undergo high-risk surgical procedures, especially those in which substantial blood loss would lead to hemodynamic instability. Now, patients are sent off to the cardiologist before every procedure including cataract or tooth extractions that carry virtually no cardiac liability. Cardiology practices can't keep up with the demand for "clearance." And when their schedules are crammed with unnecessary consultations, patients with active diseases, such as those with heart failure and coronary artery atherosclerosis, are forced to wait months to see a consultant.

Nevertheless, cardiologists and some internists continue to take referral for worthless pre-operative assessments because it is a cash cow. Patients upon whom surgeons choose to operate are usually in reasonably good physical condition; those who are very ill are declined. Consequently, most pre-operative office visits by specialists are quick and easy. Furthermore, there is the opportunity to "turn the crank" and order a variety of tests. These are usually imaging studies, performed in the office so the cardiologist can collect the technical and professional fees with a large profit margin. In many cases, imaging studies yield results that prompt further, even more expensive non-invasive testing or they land the patient in the catheterization laboratory or operating room to correct a problem they were unaware of and that didn't need treatment in the first place.

Sadly, as mentioned in the case explanation, several excellent scientific studies have proven, beyond doubt, that performing cardiac testing on an asymptomatic patient before any procedure is not helpful because discovery and treatment of latent disease does not change outcomes. In essence, this means that if a routine history and physical examination by a competent healthcare provider is negative, further evaluation is unnecessary. Carrying out corrective procedures or initiating new treatments provides no benefit and only exposes the patient to harm. An example is the prescription of beta-blockers to high-risk patients with no overt coronary artery disease. This practice was ubiquitous, and it took years for doctors to stop despite a complete lack of evidence of effectiveness in preventing post-operative cardiac events.

Despite the lack of a scientific rationale, cardiac clearance has become a big business. Large multi-specialty groups now employ their own cardiologists whose only job is to evaluate patients before procedures to assess risk and to order tests. This is an especially lucrative business for large orthopedic practices that carry out a high volume of joint replacement surgeries, for example. Nearly every patient who has a total knee or hip replacement will be seen by a cardiologist regardless of how healthy they may be, even if they are already under the care of another cardiologist. Many of these patients are scheduled to have expensive stress tests and echocardiograms before they even see the cardiologist for their initial visit. The best part for the doctors in the group practice is that this constant flow of patients for worthless testing kicks money back into everyone's pockets, each of the physicians benefitting from higher practice revenue.

For unclear reasons, medical insurance companies that, as we have seen, frequently refuse to pay for necessary medical care, unquestionably reimburse pre-operative assessments and testing, further encouraging doctors to scam the system. Insurance company tolerance for this foolishness is truly remarkable but uniform across the industry. Likewise, hospital systems that own cardiologists see no reason to stop the insanity. In fact, many of them have hired partially retired cardiologists to do cardiac clearance work, and administrators are happy when those doctors are kept busy.

In Mr. Coyle's case, the irony is that, despite an intra-practice referral system intended to generate revenue and avoid litigation, the house nevertheless came down on Drs. Wynn and Singh. Instead of carefully reviewing and dealing with the most important aspect of Mr. Coyle's case, Dr. Singh ordered a raft of worthless tests and left it to an underling to instruct the patient about stopping and starting the anticoagulant. The advice his nurse practitioner passed along was not incorrect, but it was inadequate. By not explaining the reason for caution to the patient and to Dr. Wynn, and by not documenting his instructions in the chart, Dr. Singh lost an opportunity to possibly avoid a bad outcome, and certainly to circumvent a nasty and unwinnable lawsuit.

Interrupting anticoagulation for a medical or surgical procedure is one of the most common conundrums in clinical practice. As noted in the story, anticoagulants promote bleeding. In many clinical situations, the small increase in bleeding risk does not warrant interruption of the anticoagulant. Dermatological procedures, for example, rarely require stopping an anticoagulant, especially in a patient who has an intrinsically high stroke risk.

However, if a patient is going to have a procedure in which internal bleeding is a hazard and could be life-threatening, the blood thinner must be stopped. When warfarin (Coumadin) was the most used anticoagulant, interruption was a major problem because warfarin washout and restart can take days to weeks. Many patients had to be "bridged" with heparin injections before and after their procedures to avoid blood clots and strokes.

With the advent of the new anticoagulants like Eliquis and Xarelto, interruption became easier. It takes the body only a day or two to eliminate these drugs, and only a few hours to reestablish anticoagulation. Nevertheless, for as long as the patient is off the anticoagulant, he or she is at an increased risk for having a stroke. That risk is low, less than a fraction of a percent, but it is not zero, and when a stroke occurs in this situation, it is frequently one that, like Mr. Coyle's, is life changing. Clots that come out of the left atrial appendage can be quite large and block major vessels in the brain, leading to extensive brain damage. Clot busters can help, and, in some cases, clots can be fished out with catheters. Though he regained some function, Mr. Coyle had enough of his brain damaged from lack of blood flow to be effectively and permanently disabled at a relatively young age.

CONCLUSION AND PATIENT ADVICE

The message for patients is simple: if you are instructed to have a pre-operative assessment for a common procedure, make sure you understand why. If tests are ordered, demand a rationale and plans for dealing with the results. Lean on your trusted primary care doctor to answer your questions, refuse to be ramrodded, and, if necessary, get a second opinion. There are plenty of principled specialists who continue to practice good medicine and want to do the right thing for their patients. By keeping in touch with your primary care doctor, you can also ensure good communication among the specialists who are evaluating you. Unfortunately, given the current state of medical liability and doctors' fears of being sued, and the money to be made, pre-operative "clearance" is unlikely to completely go away anytime soon.

However, the most important part of a pre-operative assessment is ascertaining what to do about medications. If you are taking cardiac drugs, especially blood thinners, make sure you understand when you should stop them and when they should be restarted. Know the risks of discontinuation and ask about your options. Finally, as all these stories have emphasized, getting your questions answered by someone you trust will inevitably pay dividends.

Story 20: Fragmentation of Care: Doctor, Who Are You Again?

"Medical mistakes are far too common because each specialist is treating (or overtreating) her own pet organ." —Allen Frances, MD

NARRATIVE

Mrs. Anders was a 79-year-old African American woman with a terrific family. She parented five children, all of whom were married with children, making for a lovely gaggle of grandchildren who doted on her endlessly. Mrs. Anders was in good health but had suffered with chronic lung disease, made worse by the secondary smoke she had inhaled for years because of her deceased husband's smoking habit. As she predicted several times during his life, the cigarettes eventually killed him, rendering Mrs. Anders a young widow. Over the many years since Mr. Anders's death, she had gotten used to living alone, knowing that her children were within easy driving distance and always available and happy to lend a hand.

Mrs. Anders also had a good primary care doctor. Dr. Orly saw her regularly and ordered laboratory testing while administering every appropriate vaccine. Dr. Orly had been particularly careful during the worst of the COVID-19 pandemic, especially given Mrs. Anders's chronic lung disease history. He made sure Mrs. Anders had all her boosters while avoiding social gatherings and crowds. When the pandemic eased, Mrs. Anders was glad to resume hosting her family for holidays and birthdays. But it was during one such celebration that she finally succumbed to the virus.

After a Sunday family dinner, several of the family members came down with COVID-19. In retrospect, one of Mrs. Anders's grandchildren remembered that a classmate had left school early the previous week with severe cold symptoms. A brief investigation revealed that the sick child did have COVID-19. Her family had not only refused to have the child vaccinated but also failed to inform the teacher or the school that their daughter was ill.

Several families caught the virus needlessly. Fortunately, most of the cases were mild.

At-home tests were positive for Mrs. Anders's sick family members, as was hers. All recovered quickly from their upper respiratory symptoms, except for Mrs. Anders. Over the next two days, her cough and fever worsened to the point that she finally called her primary care doctor for advice. He prescribed Paxlovid and instructed her to call back with an update in a few days. Mrs. Anders couldn't wait that long. By the next day she was coughing worse than ever and feeling miserable. For the first time, she was also having trouble getting her breath during any exertion.

Mrs. Anders's family came to see her and insisted she call Dr. Orly, who advised against an office visit. She was too sick for that, and it would just spread the infection among his staff. Instead, he told her that he was going to have her admitted directly to the hospital for urgent and intensive pulmonary care with the hope of keeping her off the ventilator and out of the intensive care unit. He told her that his office would call back in a few minutes with instructions.

When minutes turned into an hour, Mrs. Anders's children tired of watching her labored breathing and decided to take her to the hospital. Before they left, they called Dr. Orly's office to let him know. The secretary advised them to sit tight. Mrs. Anders's insurance company had called back and refused to allow her to be admitted unless the situation was an emergency, and their doctor talked to Dr. Orly. They had promised to get back to Dr. Orly soon, but they were still waiting.

Fortunately, Mrs. Anders's children didn't hesitate. They hung up and immediately called 911. An ambulance arrived in a few minutes and Mrs. Anders was taken to the ER of the hospital to which direct admission had been delayed. After waiting several hours in the ER, Mrs. Anders was admitted to the ICU from the ER, where her course was complicated.

Mrs. Anders received non-invasive assisted ventilation that improved her oxygenation and made her less short of breath. But what had started as a COVID-19 infection was now a rip-roaring, super-imposed bacterial pneumonia that was going to require a course of at least two and maybe three highly potent intravenous antibiotics. Fortunately, over the course of a two-week hospitalization, the pneumonia cleared, and Mrs. Anders survived, narrowly avoiding intubation and a ventilator. The infection weakened her dramatically, and she needed several days in a rehabilitation unit before she could return home to live alone. As might be expected, the transfer to the rehabilitation facility was delayed by a week, again because the insurance company required "documentation of need" before approving a brief rehab stay.

Mrs. Anders's medical adventure rattled her and her family. They were angry about all the delays in her care, and the difficulties she had to endure when very ill. They were sure that the obstacles put in place by the insurance company were directly responsible for her prolonged, and stuttering recovery from a life-threatening illness.

Her brush with death was made worse by what she later described as faceless care. To begin with, she learned that Dr. Orly no longer rounded in the hospital. The person who knew her best was out of the picture. Instead, during her long hospital course, Mrs. Anders was cared for by a legion of doctors and nurses, each of whom was polite and sympathetic but lacked the knowledge or the authority to make important management decisions.

The parade of people was impressive and included rotating hospitalists who were listed as her "attending doctors;" nocturnists who rounded in the dark, usually when she was asleep or groggy; a bevy of consultants and their fellows from at least five different departments; an army of residents, interns, and medical students who were never sure what was going on. Nevertheless, they had no compunction about asking Mrs. Anders a host of questions, most of which she didn't understand and couldn't answer. Not to forget the legion of nurses, nurses's aides, patient care technicians, laboratory personnel, housekeeping, maintenance people, and the odd chaplain who offered to pray for Mrs. Anders but didn't know her or her religious preference.

The situation would have been comical, almost like the Three Stooges movies she loved so much, but for the fact that she and her family could, under no circumstances, get straight answers from anyone about important issues. They were constantly reassured that things were going well but when it came to specific questions, like time to discharge and follow-up care and prognosis, nobody seemed to know the answers. Confusion reigned. At one point, the family received instructions about antibiotic maintenance from one specialist, only to get an entirely different answer from a hospitalist a few minutes later. Even up to the eve of her placement at a rehabilitation facility, the family wasn't sure what the plan was and what they needed to do to facilitate her physical transfer.

The other irony was that despite having a multitude of caregivers, Mrs. Anders didn't feel as if anybody was taking care of her basic needs. The only person who sat in a chair and talked to her during her hospitalization had been a third-year medical student who was practicing her interview skills. Doctors and nurses came and went at blinding speed, but Mrs. Anders wasn't taken for a walk in the hallway or given a good shower or bath. It was left to her family to take care of that business and camp out with her to help the long days go by more comfortably.

With the TV on one evening, Mrs. Anders and her youngest son could only laugh and shake their heads when a commercial for the very hospital she was sitting in appeared on the screen. With soothing piano music in the background, as it always seems to be during hospital commercials, the disembodied voice emphasized that excellent bedside care was the medical center's prime directive and that all patients would feel the love the staff would pour all over them.

Mrs. Anders was transferred to the rehabilitation facility, but the merry-go-round didn't stop. The staff had access to her EPIC chart, but they claimed that there were several missing pieces including a full list of the medications at discharge. They were also surprised by how sick she was on arrival. The hospital notes had led them to believe that she would only need a few days to get her strength back, but besides her extreme weakness, her lung problems were far from resolved. The doctors who staffed the rehab facility were not well trained in the management of lung disease, and they struggled to adjust her program to make her feel better. Consultants were not available for advice at the rehabilitation facility, except by phone. Thus, what should have been a week or so in rehab turned into a month as Mrs. Anders struggled to recover enough strength and breath to carry out her household chores.

When she finally did go home, Mrs. Anders couldn't wait to see Dr. Orly, her trusted primary care doctor. She made an appointment and appeared in his office at the end of an afternoon. She was shocked to hear from him and his staff that there had been no communication from any of her doctors at the hospital or at the rehab facility. Dr. Orly didn't have access to EPIC, the electronic medical record the hospital used, so only by reading her copy of the printed discharge instructions was he able to piece things together and figure out which medications she should be continuing. None of what he had prescribed before her hospitalization was on her new medication list. Even worse, several of her new drugs were non-generic and expensive. He knew that Mrs. Anders didn't have the resources to pay for half of them.

So, what was supposed to be a ten-minute follow-up appointment turned into an hour spent untangling the mess that had been created during Mrs. Anders's hospitalization. She was going to need frequent and involved visits over the next several weeks to which she readily assented. Anything to ensure that she wouldn't have to return to the chaos of the hospital.

The final insult was the hospital bill that came a few weeks later. It was nearly twenty pages long, listing hundreds of tests and treatments, most of which Mrs. Anders couldn't understand or identify. The list of healthcare providers who claimed they had seen her and who billed for their services was long and uncertifiable. For example, five separate doctors billed her for pulmonary consultations, and not one of the names was familiar to her or her family.

Fortunately for Mrs. Anders, her Medicare insurance was supplemented by a commercial policy she had obtained through her husband's former employer. All but a few hundred dollars of the $300,000 bill was paid by insurance at a discounted rate of $75,000, with the hospital absorbing the rest. Mrs. Anders interpreted the payment of a smaller amount as an acknowledgement that the hospital would gouge anyone foolish or disadvantaged enough to try to pay their own hospital bill.

CASE EXPLANATION

This case brings forward two monumental problems in medical care that everyone knows about but no one can solve. The first is an issue that we covered in part in an earlier story: pre-certification. In this case, the insurance company wanted the final say about directly admitting a sick patient to hospital, causing a delay that almost killed Mrs. Anders. Fortunately, Mrs. Anders's family did the right thing and called 911. Directing patients to the ER is a tactic that we use frequently to circumvent insurance company madness. This ugly problem also arises in hospital transfers. When a sick patient needs advanced management that only a few hospitals can offer, insurance companies frequently refuse the request for transfer on the premise that there is no difference in services between the referring and accepting institutions. There is no logic to such decisions. The insurance company will have to pay for hospital care somewhere, and a transfer to an institution with better facilities may facilitate the patient's recovery, thus saving money in the long run. Unless the patient expires, which is the best case scenario as far as insurance company payments are concerned.

My favorite example of pre-certification madness occurred in my practice in 1982 when we were one of only three centers in the world with access to the newly invented automatic implantable defibrillator. A hospital in Maryland had a patient in urgent need of the device. She had been resuscitated from not one but two cardiac arrests, an almost impossible piece of good fortune. Medications were ineffective in quelling her recurrent ventricular arrhythmia. We had to argue for hours with her insurance company before they begrudgingly agreed to allow the patient to come to us. Her life was saved several times by the implantable defibrillator, no thanks to the medical insurance company.

The larger and more egregious issue in Mrs. Anders's case was the fragmentation of medical care, and the extremely negative effect it had on her management and outcome. Mrs. Anders had come to rely on Dr. Orly, who had successfully managed her medical problems for many years, including stabilizing her moderately severe lung disease. She was on a good medical regimen and doing well until she was tipped over, as so many of our patients have been, by COVID-19, RSV or influenza infection.

Mrs. Anders was frightened about going to the hospital. She had heard horror stories from several of her friends about the quality of care, especially during the COVID-19 pandemic, when patients waited hours or even days to be seen and admitted to hospital, only to be placed in hallways and ignored because doctors and nurses were overwhelmed with sick patients. Most importantly, she was frightened because she would be cared for by people she didn't know or trust.

Mrs. Anders's concern was well grounded. Though the COVID-19 pandemic had waned significantly by the time she was admitted, hospitals were still being inundated with patients who had no access to primary care and therefore presented to the ER only when very ill. To make matters worse, the staffing problems increased as hospitals laid off workers, fighting hard to reverse the losses they had experienced at the peak of the pandemic. The situation was dire and exacerbated by a new way of taking care of patients, which every hospital has now adopted, and which we will discuss in the commentary: shiftwork.

Mrs. Anders eventually recovered full function and was able to enjoy her family for a few more good years. The credit for that should go to her persevering and patient primary care doctor who continued to advocate for her in every way he could. Dr. Orly spent hours of uncompensated time getting Mrs. Anders on a good medical program that she could afford and helping alter her lifestyle to make her more resilient and resistant to infections and other insults she was destined to endure.

The good doctor's reward was a disciplinary notice from the private equity firm that owned his practice. In the letter, the company let him know that his work units were disgracefully low, his revenue generation badly inadequate, and his ordering and consulting costs far above the norm. No mention was made of his outstanding patient satisfaction scores, or that he was way above the median for keeping his patients out of the hospital and the emergency room. The message was that unless he was willing to work a full day on Saturdays to bring his visit load up to par, he would be terminated. Fortunately, Dr. Orly, who had just about reached Medicare age as well as his tolerance for foolishness, had a wealthy spouse. He was not unhappy to say goodbye to his clinical practice. His patients and staff, who adored him, were not as sanguine.

COMMENTARY

In bygone days, doctors and their trainees admitted patients to the hospital on schedule or through the emergency room with the expectation that they would be responsible for that specific patient's care for the duration of their hospitalization. Physicians would round daily on their patients and cover them when they were on call. It was at times a grueling task to be available nearly continuously, but the benefit was that the patients were well cared for. Management was seamless, coordinated by a doctor who knew the case and the patient well. The patients knew who their doctors were, especially since their private doctor was usually their hospital attending physician. Specialists who consulted on hospitalized patients were expected to communicate directly with the attending physician and the house staff immediately after they saw the patient. They could make recommendations, but orders could only be written by the attending physician or their designate.

Residents and interns assigned to specific patients were expected to know everything about each one, to brief the attending doctors on a regular basis, and to round with the resident team every day. Nurses and their assistants were an essential part of the team, assigned to the same patients each day, caring for all their needs and providing reassurance. They were expected to have a good grasp of the patient's problems so they could answer questions quickly and intelligently.

The best thing about this traditional system is that everyone knew who was in charge and responsible. While residents, nurses and students were vital members of the care team and contributed to the daily care of the patients, it was the attending physician who called the shots and made decisions based on her knowledge, experience and consultation with other senior doctors. The attending physician rounded daily and was continually briefed on the status of her patients. In a crisis, it was the attending physician who decided what urgent steps needed to be taken, based on her knowledge of the disease and her familiarity with the patient and her family.

Three developments unraveled this system, which had worked so well for patients and doctors for so many years. First, primary care doctors became so busy with their practices that they no longer had time to round in the hospital and take calls from nurses and house staff. They had to hurry through patient rounds and there were long delays in responding to urgent calls which, as in Mrs. Anders's case, necessitated a frantic trip to the ER.

Witnessing a sharp decline in the quality of care that this abandonment caused, hospitals decided to hire hospitalists, usually young and inexperienced physicians who would spend their entire day on the hospital floors and in the intensive care units, their only job being to take care of hospitalized patients. To make the job palatable, they instituted shift work whereby physicians would work for eight to twelve hours and then hand their patients off to another doctor. Alternating day and night shifts was grueling and unpopular, so nocturnists were invented, doctors who worked only the night shift but were paid a sharp hourly premium. Some hospitals taxed primary care physicians to pay the high costs of hospitalist coverage.

Communication among the many hospitalists and nocturnists became ever more difficult as their numbers grew and their associations became more tenuous. Hospitalists were discouraged from signing out patients to the next shift by phone or in person, and encouraged to use the EMR as the message carrier. Some even advocated using artificial intelligence to bridge care between practitioners, a message that boils the blood of any seasoned clinician.

Next, medical educators became convinced that interns and residents were working too hard and not getting enough sleep. A few famous cases of intern error had ignited a media firestorm. Accrediting agencies began to insist on hour limits for house staff. Now, instead of having a resident in the house who knew the patients, admitting them to the hospital and rounding on them every day, trainees worked shifts and passed patients on, just like the hospitalists. As we have discussed previously, when eventually examined in properly performed trials years after the work hour rules went into effect, resident rest had absolutely no impact on clinical outcomes. The on-call system that had worked for decades had been dismantled based on unproven opinions and hearsay and for no good reason.

I distinctly remember the great frustration of attempting to communicate with house staff when I rounded on patients in the hospital. Inevitably, house staff weren't on the floor, usually off attending a conference or flailing away at a research project, which, discussed in another vignette, added little or nothing to medical knowledge. Worse, I couldn't figure out which resident was responsible for my patient, and neither could the nurses or other personnel on the floor.

Finally, nursing positions were slashed to save money. In the place of these more expensive healthcare providers, hospitals hired various assistants who were trained to do a few tasks but were unable to truly care for the patients. Nurses were charged with overseeing care on hospital floors but were assigned so many more patients that it was impossible for them to learn who the patients were, let alone help them with their problems and provide any measure of comfort. Unlike their workload, salaries for nurses did not increase, leading to an exodus from the profession, unionization and job actions.

The result of these changes in the medical care delivery model was a dramatic deterioration in the quality of hospital care. Patients and their families were no longer able to identify their caregivers and felt helpless and poorly informed. Common problems that used to be addressed easily now mushroomed into disasters. Mistakes like administering the wrong drug or the wrong dose or taking out the healthy organ increased to the point that even legislators took notice and started passing legislation to improve transparency. But most of these measures compounded the complexity of care, solving nothing. Post-discharge care became particularly difficult with frequent omission of necessary medications or needless continuation of dangerous therapies caused by lack of communication during patient hand-offs.

Is there a way to put the broken system back together? It seems unlikely. Increasing use of faceless technology and progressive sub-specialization virtually guarantees that patients will be treated even more like commodities than human beings. They almost must be. Thanks to hospital closures and unavailability of primary care physicians, the sheer number of patients who are visiting emergency rooms and being admitted for serious disease has become unmanageable. Delivering individual and personal care to the multitudes is simply impossible when scores of patients are sitting in hallways waiting for hospital bed assignments.

Hospital television advertisements notwithstanding, compassionate care is now a luxury that only a few can afford. Hiring a concierge physician is a strategy that may work for the wealthy by paying a doctor to be available in an emergency, and, best of all, to coordinate care. Hospitals now take pride in having "luxury suites" for rich people who not only want better food and silk sheets, but more attentive caregivers. If you can shell out a few thousand dollars, you will have private nurses and attendants who will know everything about you and answer all your questions. Some hospitals advertise "nurse navigators" to shepherd the elderly and impaired, many of whom volunteer from the community. But the deluge of sick patients and liability concerns has caused most of those programs to curtail their activity or shut down altogether.

For most patients, navigating through a piecemeal and broken healthcare system will be a challenge of increasing magnitude. Relying on the availability of family members or good friends may be the best solution. Hospitals have increasingly installed day beds in patient rooms, unwittingly acknowledging that a caregiver would be wise to remain in the hospital overnight to help when staff levels are unconscionably low, and hours go by until a call bell is answered.

The ultimate solution to the hospital care crisis would be to better fund acute care hospitals and to increase the number of intermediate care facilities so that patients can get the therapy they need. This would obviously entail redirecting money that is currently wasted on legions of hospital administrators, worthless testing, unnecessary procedures, and bogus treatments to where it is truly needed. Our legislative leaders refuse to make the necessary sweeping changes mainly because of intense lobbying by corporations and plaintiff malpractice attorneys who know that there are billions more to be milked out of the bloated, dysfunctional medical system, and angry and frustrated patients.

CONCLUSION

It is axiomatic that patients want, need and deserve holistic and compassionate care. The complexity of modern medicine challenges that priority. It is simply not possible for an individual physician or nurse to meet all her patient's needs. Consultants, assistant nurses and house officers are crucially necessary. The main challenge is to organize the medical care team to maintain continuity of care. Fragmentation for any reason is a formula for disaster. This is not the fault of the caregivers. Most of them care deeply about the patient they are treating and want to deliver the best care. It is the system that defeats them.

Physicians who, in the past, sacrificed their private lives to their profession are no longer willing to do so. In many ways, this is a good development. Healthcare providers who are well rounded and happy with their private lives are less susceptible to burnout and more likely to persevere and to remain in practice longer. However, I fear that the pendulum has swung too far in the other direction. Young physicians are no longer held to high standard. They expect to work their shifts and leave their patients' problems to someone else, no matter how ill, when their shift is up. Correcting or disciplining a house officer is cause for reprimand for "attending physician bullying" and so their mistakes are perpetuated.

Residents and hospitalists pay little attention to the complexity of handoffs and lack either the time or the sensibility to share with the next shift worker what might be the most important facts about their patients. They also expect to tap the expertise of multiple specialists and to cede responsibility and decision making to a bevy of consultants. While this increases expertise, it creates havoc for the patients. Like Mrs. Anders, patients feel disconnected and overwhelmed, unable to identify decision makers and key caregivers.

PATIENT ADVICE

Once again, a knowledgeable patient has a better chance of navigating through a serious illness. In Mrs. Anders's case, her family was supportive and helpful in getting answers, but her primary care doctor was her most important anchor. Unfortunately, and to Mrs. Anders's chagrin, his old way of practicing medicine was not sustainable. Like many others of his generation, he preferred to leave medicine rather than tow the profit line.

It is not unreasonable to anticipate many of the issues I have raised and to be prepared to take responsibility for your care. Finding out who is supposed to be in charge and making sure that person is responsive to your needs is paramount. However, it is important not to have unrealistic expectations. Medicine is not and never again will be practiced in the way that attracted many, like me, to the profession. Remember Dr. Lown's advice to sit down in the patient's presence, to make the patient believe theirs was the most important case on the floor, and as such, deserving of our undivided attention? Now, when was the last time you saw a doctor do that?

My Overall Conclusion

"Healing is dealing with what is not statistical, what is not generalizable in the way science generalizes. It confronts the fact that every human being is different in so many ways." —Bernard Lown, MD

It is abundantly clear that medicine, once practiced as an honorable profession by highly principled people, is in jeopardy. The profession that focused on treating and healing the whole patient has been eclipsed by the new paradigm of revenue production. Once medicine started generating big money (literally, trillions of dollars), it was only a matter of time before our profession would be contaminated. The perpetrators included hospital administrators, insurance company executives, drug company owners, private equity/venture capital opportunists, accrediting bodies, professional organizations, regulatory bodies, and hosts of others. Medicine would no longer be owned and operated by physicians but taken over by people who didn't take an oath to protect patients, and who don't understand the physician's core mission: to be the patient's ombudsman, charged with caring for patients with serious illnesses with total dedication and an abundance of compassion. In short, to listen and then to heal.

The people to whom doctors ceded control of hospitals, practices, payment, regulation, and product development have focused on the things they do understand: how to gain control of organizations, generate large revenue, reward their stockholders, and secure and maintain their lucrative positions. They replicate and propagate while they convince their constituents that without them, the system would collapse. They cleverly influence local and state governments to manufacture regulations that they profess are for the good of the patient, but which are rarely proven to cause better outcomes. Accrediting organizations visit our hospitals and look for violations so that they can justify their existence. I was flabbergasted when I learned that a hospital was cited after a first-year, stressed-out resident, trying to take care of her patients, was highjacked by a site visitor. The resident was ordered to answer a question about crisis response she was supposed to have learned during hours of computer-based training. When queried, the harried resident couldn't recite the five things to do when an active shooter is in the building. She could only think of one: "run like hell."

The rules of operation that are laid out by accrediting bodies also provide a rationale to hire even more administrators to overcome the ultimate threat of loss of certification, which rarely ever happens. And what if that threat was carried out and a busy hospital was shuttered by an accreditor? Think about trying to close a large busy hospital because a trash can wasn't emptied.

Administrators generate no revenue themselves but pay themselves enormous salaries that, in a rational world, could never be justified. They are incentivized, but bonuses are not based on quality of care but on financial performance. How else could the CEO of a failed healthcare system receive a multi-million-dollar buyout while the hospitals he ran literally closed their doors? CEOs remain in control by stacking their boards with businesspeople who are even more money-motivated than they, and who have little or no knowledge of healthcare or how best to deliver it. To pretend that they respect practitioners, they throw bones to them on occasions like Nurses or Doctors Day, assuming that the practitioner minions will be grateful for a cold scrambled egg and bacon breakfast in the hospital cafeteria, and a lapel flower.

What we now have is massively misdirected spending. The trillions we spend on healthcare in the US has landed us at the very bottom of quality among developed countries using any metric you choose. This disconnect is not hard to decipher. Ask yourself how many nurses, the people who really take care of patients, could a hospital hire if they didn't pay a seven or eight figure salary to a drone who sits in a corporate office all day twiddling her thumbs? How much cheaper could medicines be if we eliminated or restricted Pharmacy Benefits Managers? How much less expensive would health insurance premiums be if we shed a dozen or so insurance company vice presidents or restricted their ability to advertise on television or with giant insignia in baseball stadiums and hockey arenas? The examples of waste are legion and unique to our country, where capitalism rules. The possibilities for healthcare improvement with reappropriation of funds are astounding.

It should come as no surprise that nearly two-thirds of Americans no longer trust the healthcare system or its ability to deal with common diseases. Likewise, the public has sunk into a mire of confusion about so many important medical issues. Thanks to the font of misinformation we call the internet, our patients are now chock full of wrong ideas. It usually takes me as long during office visits to disabuse patients of false notions as it does to teach them what is true. Marty Makary, the new FDA Commissioner, in his book *Blind Spots* describes dozens of falsehoods that continue to circulate and interfere with delivery of good medical care. From the idea that hormone replacement therapy causes breast cancer to breakfast being the most important meal of the day, to the eggs raise cholesterol misunderstandings, Dr. Makarey points out where the messages to the public went wrong and who was responsible. In nearly every case, the critical factor that kept falsehoods alive was greed.

Stubborn adherence to debunked and overcooked theories is de rigueur in medicine, perpetuated by large professional organizations, misdirected regulatory agencies, and powerful academics who struggle to maintain their stranglehold on medical practice through practice guidelines and algorithms that are not entirely evidence based. How else to explain the absurdities of labelling opioids as non-addictive, abandoning silicone breast implants for reconstructive mammoplasties, denying that HIV could be transmitted via blood transfusions, pronouncing the harmlessness of marijuana, proscribing eggs to lower serum cholesterol, restricting hormone replacement therapy to prevent breast cancer, or mandating surgery for all cases of appendicitis. How about guideline committees abandoning LDL-cholesterol, arguably the best surrogate for cardiovascular outcomes, as the most important metric in making decisions about whether to prescribe a statin to at-risk patients. In each of these examples, good clinical trial data were pushed aside in favor of popular beliefs, widely held opinion, and foolish stubbornness

Ironically, our call to action has elicited a response from politicians that may not be at all helpful. The current administration has made it clear that it intends to be disruptive to correct what it perceives to be "corruption" within our current healthcare system. While this book substantiates some of their claims, and their intentions may be good, the draconian measures they have proposed will do little to cure the ills of the system. Consider the impact of repealing the Affordable Care Act and cutting Medicaid on accessibility to care for the disadvantaged. Shifting power to insurance conglomerates and pharmaceutical giants will increase the cost of care and limit access across the board. Our ability to insure patients with "pre-existing conditions" is vital to maintaining their health, but that provision is in deep jeopardy.

Appointing incompetent bureaucrats to run cabinet-level departments will jeopardize the integrity of important regulatory agencies such as the Food and Drug Administration, the Centers for Disease Control, and the National Institutes of Health, placing all of us at risk of preventable diseases. Deporting employed immigrants and limiting ingress of skilled healthcare workers will exacerbate an already critical shortage. Imposing exorbitant tariffs will choke the fragile medical product supply chain. Interrupting funding for research will retard the development of important new therapeutics. In short, attempting to fix the system with sweeping changes that are improperly motivated and ill-conceived will make the things I warn about in this book exponentially worse.

The anti-vax movement may be the most dangerous of the lies that have been put forward by politicians and circulated on social media. A few vocal miscreants with little or no medical knowledge have convinced a sizeable percentage of patients and parents that vaccines are not only unnecessary, but harmful. The allegation that vaccines cause autism is not supported by a multitude of well-performed clinical trials. Vaccine skepticism is even more difficult to understand given the fact that the COVID-19 pandemic was halted only when enough people were vaccinated to bring us to the point of population immunity. Mandating placebo-controlled trials of new vaccines to treat dangerous diseases for which safe and effective therapy is already available is not only scientifically suspect but ethically bankrupt.

With fewer children and adults vaccinated against common diseases, it will only be a matter of time until disease outbreaks savage schools, kill and disable children, and push the already terribly stressed healthcare system to the brink. Measles is but the first example of previously vanquished diseases that will rear their ugly heads again. A resurgence of polio is almost unimaginable but entirely possible in an under-vaccinated world.

Given our current situation, which is unlikely to change for the foreseeable future, it is incumbent upon patients to look out for themselves and for each other. To do so, they need to be armed with as much information about the healthcare system and their diseases as possible. This book is my attempt to advise patients as to some of the major hazards that exist in the modern medical care nightmare. As we have seen, there are many mines to avoid in the minefield, some of them extremely well hidden but highly lethal if stepped on. The commonality is patient exploitation for the sake of profit.

As we have learned from so many of life's misfortunes, it you want to find the perpetrator of or the rationale for deadly deeds, follow the money.

Any physician or other healthcare provider who reads this book will recognize the truth of what I have asserted. They will identify with my frustration at seeing thousands of undaunted and underappreciated practitioners continue to sacrifice their private lives to make sure that patients are well cared for. Some may even opine that I have underestimated the crisis by not covering all the ills that afflict our healthcare system, and they have a point. One of the problems I encountered in writing this book is that, daily, I read about a new issue that I wanted to expound upon. Colleagues, upon hearing about the book, were anxious to regale me with stories of how the healthcare system had failed them and their patients. The situation is clearly desperate and becoming more so every day.

It appears unlikely that doctors at any level, including our professional organizations, are going to be able to affect change in the current paradigm. There is simply too much money invested in maintaining the status quo. Legislators are loathe to defy the multi-billion-dollar insurance industry or lawyer lobbies that fund their campaigns and line their pockets. Like so many of our largest societal problems such as gun control, the environment, homelessness, and poverty, it will take a revolution to change course and restore our ability to truly care for the sick and dying the way we want to. However, staying strong and uncompromising when it comes to taking care of individual patients remains our sacred charge. Physicians also need to look for opportunities to partner with their patients, to make them aware of the plight of healthcare providers and to encourage them to agitate for change. United, doctors and patients have a much better chance of breaking through the glass ceiling and getting legislators at the state and local level to do the right thing.

Doctors also need to police themselves. We know that there is a small percentage of physicians who practice bad medicine, deliberately gaming the system at the expense of their patients. There are few mechanisms available to investigate these doctors, to revoke their licenses, or to prosecute them in criminal court. State medical societies and our professional organizations need to become proactive in this regard to make our profession less vulnerable to bad publicity and loss of public trust.

To survive the current crisis and to effect change, practitioners also need each other. We take solace in knowing that good doctors and nurses share an unwavering commitment to preserve the health and the dignity of our patients. Alice Chen and Vivek Murthy in a recent *New England Journal of Medicine* perspective said it perfectly: "This is a time for us to reach out and support each other—to check on each other, listen to each other…We can remind each other that we are not alone."

As for our patients, they may be able to navigate the system, albeit it with great expenditures of time and energy. Many of my retired patients have told me that accessing healthcare and going to doctor appointments is their new full-time job. Estimates are that the average Medicare patient spends the equivalent of three work weeks per year accessing medical care, much of which they probably don't even need.

A significant portion of wasted time is spent online or on the phone trying to get through to medical offices just to make an appointment. One of my friends and patients spent a beautiful day in May on the phone, trying to get an endocrinology appointment for his wife who was a newly diagnosed diabetic. All the practices he contacted quoted at least a four-month wait, a problem because their primary care doctor had emphasized the importance of initiating treatment promptly. My friend was overjoyed when a university hospital practice told him that they could easily fit her in for a June 10th appointment. When he looked at his calendar, he saw that the date fell on a Sunday. It turned out that the appointment he was being offered was on a Monday morning, thirteen months hence.

But no matter how smart they are, how hard they try, and how much time they devote to the task of obtaining and sustaining good medical care, patients will always need the help of a sympathetic and dedicated healthcare provider, preferably a generalist. They will also benefit from the honest advice of people they know who work in medicine, who have a brain and a heart, and are wise enough not to step beyond their expertise. Tapping the wisdom of friends or relatives who are or were healthcare providers and have familiarity with the system is another good way of accessing accurate and appropriate information. I find myself in that role with increasing frequency, as the insanity of the medical care system reaches new heights. With increasing frustration, I attempt to lay out a reasonable path of care for friends and family, all the time knowing that the odds of penetrating the madness to attain a truly good outcome shrink with every passing year.

The challenge for all of us as patients is to find the precious purveyors of truth, ask them questions, which they are usually happy to address, and believe and rely on their learned answers. They may not always be entirely correct, but discourse with them will start you on a path to a good outcome.

And when, with much good fortune and maybe even divine intervention, patients identify an oracle, someone they can trust and whom they understand, someone who patiently answers their questions no matter how mundane, and who really cares about their welfare, they need to hold on to that person, literally for dear life.

ACKNOWLEDGMENTS

I am indebted to the many people who impacted my career and inspired this book. It would be impossible to list all of them. Drs. Barbara Roberts and Bernard Lown lead the list, as you have seen, but I will call out a few others. Dr. Sidney Wolfe and I collaborated on several projects early in my academic career, including a groundbreaking study of unnecessary pacemaker implantation that led to my appearance at a Senate Subcommittee meeting. Frequently scorned by mainstream medicine, Sid was a gadfly who dedicated his life to patient advocacy and never compromised. He inspired me to speak out.

Dr. Raymond Lipicky was the director of the Cardiorenal Division of the FDA when I joined its advisory committee. Ray lived the Oliver Wendell Holmes quotation, "I am not a therapeutic nihilist but a therapeutic skeptic." No one in medicine taught people how to put aside bias and to seek the truth in a data set better than Ray. His influence on medicine will live on for generations.

Drs. Richard Verrier and Philip Podrid provided me with so much of my early experimental and clinical training and patiently mentored me as I matured into an independent investigator. They remain close friends.

James Kaufmann, PhD is my editor and has been throughout my writing career. Jim and I went to high school together and, though our paths have diverged, our sensibilities remain in lockstep. In addition to his brilliant technical work, Jim's advice about content has been spot on and has been essential to the success of all my books.

Nancy Fullam is also a close friend and a former law partner of my wife, Dorothy. Nancy has read my books pre-publication to be doubly certain that I have not stepped on anybody's toes inadvertently. Like Jim, her comments about content were concise and invaluable.

Naomi Rosenblatt is my publisher and from the beginning has advocated for a book that tells the truth about the plight of our medical care system and how patients can avoid its pitfalls. I have learned a great deal from Naomi, from my energetic publicists Deb Kohan and Aric Cohen, and from my social media guru Kristin Jensen. Ken Kraft and David Gechman at River Knoll Productions have helped me transmit my ideas to screen and have done so with patience and skill.

Donna Simonds is and has been my administrative assistant for over forty years and has been instrumental in keeping me on schedule and in line. She and my other assistant, Roe Wells, have been my "secret weapons" and both have become cherished members of our family.

My wife Dorothy, our three daughters, Susan, Jaime, and Olivia, and their spouses have shaped my wisdom about so many things and helped me gather the courage to speak out about many important issues. I treasure their support and love.

I have trained hundreds of cardiologists and arrhythmia specialists during my career. I am indebted to them for carrying on the tradition of caring medicine, passed on to me by my mentors.

Finally, I want to thank my patients. The stories in this book are based on their journeys. Each person I have cared for has inspired me and challenged me to be a better physician and human being. I hope I haven't let you down.

GLOSSARY

Ablation: Procedure in which cardiac tissue is destroyed using energy (usually thermal) that is delivered through catheters threaded through blood vessels to the heart. The most common application is to eliminate fast heart rhythms.

Administrative Harm: Damage to patients, practitioners and healthcare facilities by administrator mistakes or misjudgments.

Aneurysm: weakness in the wall of a blood vessel, usually an artery.

Atrial fibrillation: Lack of an organized rhythm in the upper chambers of the heart that may cause palpitations, shortness or breath and a stroke if clots leave the non-functioning atrium and travel to the brain.

Aortic stenosis: Blockage of the main heart valve that allows blood to leave the heart and travel to the general circulation.

Arrhythmia: A general term to describe anytime the heart is out of rhythm. It includes skipped beats, fast and slow heart rhythms, and sustained events that require an intervention for termination.

Blood thinners: Drugs which prevent coagulation of blood. They can be used for multiple purposes including prevention of stroke in atrial fibrillation. Heparin and warfarin are older drugs while the direct acting oral anticoagulants (DOACs) have become available more recently and may be safer and more effective for some patients and indications.

Calcium Score: An imaging technique to quantify the amount of calcium that is contained in the blood vessels that supply blood to the heart. Higher scores mean a greater probability of an arterial blockage.

CAT scan: A test in which an internal organ like the heart is imaged in several dimensions yielding a detailed view and reconstruction of the organ's anatomy.

Cardiac Catheterization: A test in which catheters are inserted into the heart through peripheral blood vessels. Dye can be injected to allow the vessels to be precisely imaged. If blockages are found, they can be opened with a balloon and a stent. This procedure is called a PCI (percutaneous coronary intervention).

Cardiac arrest: The sudden loss of the heart's rhythm causing blood to stop flowing to the body's organs.

Carotid artery: Those arteries in the neck that carry blood to the brain. Blockage of these arteries is the most common reason for a stroke.

DVT/PE (deep vein thrombosis/pulmonary embolism): Clots form in the veins of the leg that cause leg swelling and pain. If those clots are released from the veins, they may travel to the lungs and cause loss of oxygenation of the blood and death. Air or fat introduced into the circulation by mistake can also travel to the lungs with a similar outcome.

Defibrillator: A device that delivers a large amount of electrical energy to the heart to place it back in rhythm after a cardiac arrest. These devices can be used externally, or they can be implanted to function automatically.

EMR (electronic medical record): A computerized record that stores comprehensive patient information available to a variety of caregivers and payers.

Generic drugs: Copies of drugs usually manufactured at a lower price but with equivalent efficacy and safety.

Hernia: A weakness in a structure such as a muscle or tendon that is supposed to enclose an internal body part like a bowel.

Heart attack: Layman's term for a myocardial infarction. Closure of an artery that supplies blood to the heart resulting in damage to the heart muscle.

Internship/Residency/Fellowship: Periods of medical training after medical school during which physicians acquire skills in specific specialties.

Medicare Advantage: A plan in which an insurance company receives Medicare funds directly from the government and disperses them along with a purchased supplement to pay for specific procedures for clients.

MBC (metastatic breast cancer): A term to describe breast cancer that has spread outside of the breast to distant organs like bone and brain.

MRI (magnetic resonance imaging): An imaging technique using magnets that, like CAT scans, allows for a detailed look at internal organs.

Migraine headache: A severe form of headache caused by spasm of arteries that supply blood to the brain.

Nurse Practitioners/Physician Assistants: Healthcare providers who are trained to administer medical care at an advanced level under the supervision of a physician. Training and responsibilities for both these groups of physician extenders are similar.

Prior authorization or precertification: The process of obtaining a guarantee of payment from an insurance company for a specific treatment or procedure.

Stroke: Damage to the brain caused by interruption of blood flow or by bleeding into the brain substance.

Surgical clearance: The process by which a healthcare provider is asked to assess the suitability of a patient for a surgical procedure.

AUTHOR BIO

Dr. Peter Kowey is Professor of Medicine and Clinical Pharmacology at Thomas Jefferson University, Emeritus Chief of the Division of Cardiovascular Diseases at the Lankenau Heart Institute, and the William Wikoff Smith Chair in Cardiovascular Research at the Lankenau Institute for Medical Research.

Dr. Kowey is an internationally recognized expert in heart rhythm disorders. His research, regulatory and clinical trial expertise, and industry consultations have led to the development of innovative therapies for cardiac arrhythmias. Dr Kowey is the recipient of over 150 grants, has written over 450 papers and scientific reports, and has co-edited 5 textbooks on cardiac arrhythmia. He has trained hundreds of fellows who practice cardiology and cardiac electrophysiology around the world.

Dr. Kowey is a Fellow of the American Heart Association, the American College of Cardiology, the American College of Physicians and the Heart Rhythm Society and several other professional organizations. He was a member of the Cardio-Renal Drug Advisory Committee and the Cardiovascular Devices Advisory Committee of the Food and Drug Administration. Dr. Kowey has been the recipient of numerous awards including the Edward S. Cooper Award from the American Heart Association, and the William Osler Award from the University of Miami.

Dr. Kowey is a graduate of St. Joseph's University (and served on the university's Board of Trustees) and the University of Pennsylvania School of Medicine. He completed his residency training in internal medicine at Penn State University and was a fellow in cardiovascular medicine and research at the Harvard University School of Public Health, the Peter Bent Brigham Hospital, and the West Roxbury VA Hospital. He has published five medical mystery novels over the last fifteen years. Dr. Kowey and his wife, Dorothy, live with their Portuguese water dogs in Bryn Mawr and the Pocono Mountains and have three attorney daughters and six grandchildren.

www.ingramcontent.com/pod-product-compliance
Lightning Source LLC
LaVergne TN
LVHW050333141025
823427LV00038B/371